Dr. Nooshin Khoshkhesal Darvish

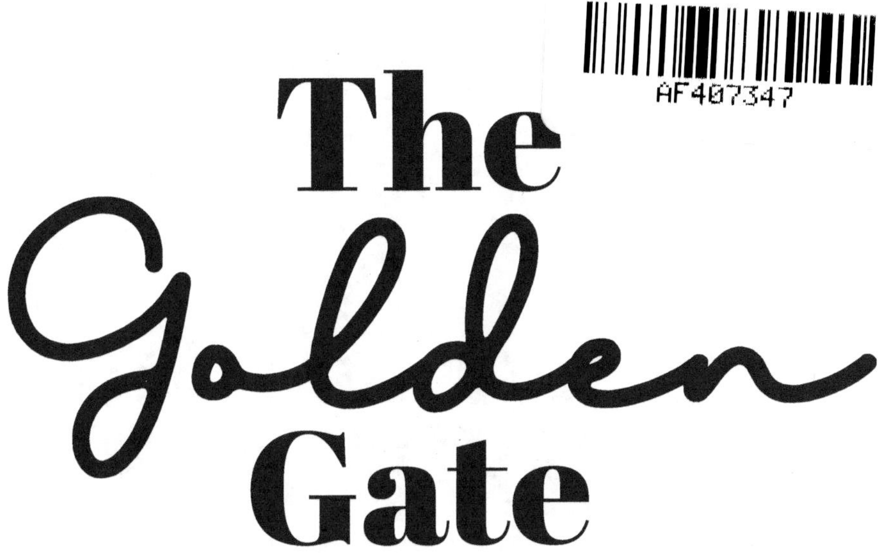

The Golden Gate

Unleash Your Feminine Powers to Graceful Aging

A GUIDE TO LIVING LONGER AND HEALTHIER WITH JOY

PRAISE FOR THE GOLDEN GATE

In the amazing book, *The Golden Gate: Unleash Your Feminine Powers to Graceful Aging* by Dr. Nooshin K. Darvish, we are invited to enter a game-changer for women's vitalistic living. Through her KHOSH Method™, Dr. Darvish helps us tap into our power to heal ourselves and the world around us. I had the privilege of experiencing this method alongside other women in a transformative journey, where we shed our pain, doubts, and traumas and emerged more robust and healthier.

In *The Golden Gate*, Dr. Darvish encourages us to embrace all aspects of ourselves, laugh through our generational wounds, and remove the veil of disease through the wisdom of healing. Her work is truly miraculous; the book is a testament to her expertise and passion.

Words cannot describe the miraculous nature of Dr. Darvish's work and how she captivates all of us in the beauty of who we are and what it means to enter the Golden Gate and the profound wisdom for us all.

The Golden Gate is a must-read if you want to release and rejuvenate, move beyond society's beliefs about aging, and step into your power. I am alive today because of Dr. Darvish's work, and I know countless other women who have benefited tremendously from her holistic approach to healing. This is not just a book to read. It is a book to live by!

Dr. Pat Baccili, PhD
Owner & Founder, The Transformation Network
Founder, Voices in Empowering Women

Empowered women and girls are in fact the Golden Gates to sustainable development. "Educate a girl, and transform a village," is immutable because as women we pay it forward, and positive change multiplies. *The Golden Gate: Unleash Your Feminine Powers to Graceful Aging* highlights finding our healthy and resilient selves, mind, body, and soul, to rise as a phoenix rises from the ashes of the past, to realize our full selves and transform for the better our own village.

Mahnaz Aflatooni Javid, Ed.D
CEO & President, Mona Foundation

The Golden Gate is not merely a superficial cosmetic enhancement of existing paradigms; it is a deep dive into the individual terrains of each woman. Dr. Darvish emphasizes the fundamental importance of understanding and assessing the unique landscape of every woman. It is a departure of the one-size-fits-all approaches and commitment to addressing the core issues rather than superficial symptoms.

The Golden Gate: Unleash Your Feminine Powers to Graceful Aging is more than a book – it is a guide, a beacon, and a clarion call for women to reclaim their power, embrace their authenticity, and lead others through the Golden Gates within. Dr. Darvish's passion, wisdom, and transformative energy echo through every page, inviting women to embark on a journey of self-discovery, empowerment, and holistic wellbeing.

Nasha Winters, ND, FABNO
Executive Director of the Metabolic Terrain Institute of Health
Author: "The Metabolic Approach to Cancer" and "Mistletoe and the Emerging Future of Integrative Oncology"

Dr. Darvish's book, *The Golden Gate*, is a definitive guide to women's health and an unabashing call for action to all women (and their men!) to reclaim their power and transform their lives and the world around them from within!

Her inspiring life story and the medical insights she shares of those of her patients and the six-step KHOSH Method™ are powerful reminders that the greatest joy comes from living a holistic life of service to others... the more you give to the world around you the more comes back to you in joy and good health... and this service-oriented mindset is the secret to graceful aging! A landmark book every woman should read... men may find it revealing too!

Shiva Dustdar
Dean of the EIB Institute,
Director of the European Investment Bank (EIB), Luxembourg

Dr. Darvish's book, *The Golden Gate*, is a captivating journey through the realms of mind, soul, and body. As I delved into its pages, I couldn't help but appreciate the meticulous organization and insightful content that it offers to women seeking a holistic approach to aging gracefully.

The book begins with a powerful introduction that sets the tone for what lies ahead. Dr. Darvish skillfully guides readers through a series of thought-provoking chapters, each addressing a crucial aspect of a woman's life. From the nuances of being a woman in today's world to navigating the dance of duality, the author covers a wide range of topics with depth and wisdom.

In Dr. Darvish's signature style, *The Golden Gate* is not just a book; it's a holistic journey that intertwines scientific knowledge with spiritual wisdom. Dr. Darvish's ability to communicate complex ideas in an accessible manner makes this book a valuable resource for women of all ages.

Whether you are navigating the challenges of hormonal changes or seeking a roadmap for graceful aging, Dr. Darvish's insights will undoubtedly resonate with you. This book is a testament to the author's dedication to empowering women to unleash their feminine power and embrace the golden years with grace. Bravo!!

Jessica Peatross, MD, GP

Founder, Wellness Plus

Dr. Nooshin K. Darvish's *The Golden Gate: Unleash Your Feminine Powers to Graceful Aging* is a transformative guide that empowers women to embrace aging with grace and wisdom. Merging her profound medical knowledge with personal insights, Darvish offers a holistic approach to womanhood and wellbeing. Her innovative KHOSH Method™ provides practical steps for balancing and rejuvenating the mind, body, and spirit to create joy and longevity. This book is an essential read for women of all ages seeking to enrich their journey through life's stages with dignity and joy.

Dr. Roy Steiner
Senior Vice President, The Rockefeller Foundation

Dedicated to My Dearest Mother,
Nahid Varqai Mazkouri Khoshkhesal,
and to all the women who came before her,
and to all the women who come after her.

I Love You,
I Honor You,
and I Am Grateful to You!

Yá Bahá'u'l-Abhá!
O Thou Glory of the All-Glorious

THE GOLDEN GATE

Dr. Nooshin Khoshkhesal Darvish

Edited and published by The Boss Books/Libri d'Impresa Edizioni

One Hour Marketing Srl
Via Torino 9, 21013 – Gallarate (VA), Italy
www.thebossbooks.com

ISBN 9791280622891

Contents

"To walk where
there is no path,
To breathe where
there is no air,
To see where
there is no light –
This is Faith."

Ruhiyyih Khanum
(Mary Maxwell)

FOREWORD

In the labyrinth of life, there are individuals whose paths resonate so deeply with ours that their journey becomes intertwined with our own. Though I have yet to meet Dr. Nooshin K. Darvish in person, our parallel trajectories, shared philosophies, and profound dedication to the empowerment of women have forged a connection that transcends physical encounters. As I delve into the pages of her transformative book, *The Golden Gate: Unleash Your Feminine Powers to Graceful Aging*, I am compelled to amplify its significance and declare a resounding call to action – a call for women to reclaim their essence, to traverse the Golden Gates within themselves, and to illuminate the way for others to do the same.

Dr. Darvish's work is more than a book; it is a manifesto for a new era of femininity and women's power. In a world that often attempts to confine women to predefined roles and takes the liberty to impose an unrealistic and unobtainable level of perfection, this book serves as a guiding light, inviting women to step up through the gates of their own potential, transcending limitations, and societal expectations.

For years I was an assistant professor in a sociology course at my local college, dedicated to unraveling the intricacies of women's health, and was always shocked to find most of the students I encountered lacked a fundamental understanding of their own bodies.

This lack of awareness viewed women's natural life and monthly cycles as abnormal, needing medical intervention.

Dr. Darvish's book delves into the core of such misconceptions, unveiling the intricacies of the female body and mind. It is a journey through the three generations that exist within each woman – maiden, the mother, and the wise woman. This triad encapsulates the essence of the female experience, an experience that continues to be misunderstood and undermined.

In the current phase of my own life, I am saddened to see my peers perceive menopause as a disease to be feared rather than a transformative phase to be revered. Dr. Darvish challenges this paradigm, asserting that menopause is not a state of dis-ease, but a terrain issue, as much as a state of mind. It is a gate that beckons women to rediscover and recreate themselves, much like the gates of menarche, fertility, and perimenopause invite the same.

The narrative in *The Golden Gate* extends beyond biology, touching upon culture, gender, humanity – even the influence of corporations and industry-driven paradigms. Dr. Darvish eloquently explores the multifaceted abilities of women – the ability to multitask, create community, lead, and protect. She makes me think of one of my colleagues, Dr. Kayla Osterhoff, a neuropsychophysiologist and renowned women's health expert who is pioneering research and innovations that are changing the landscape of feminine health. Celebrating the inherent differences between female and male brains is a key to unlocking our true potential.

A poignant and personal story shared in the book is that of Dr. Darvish's own mother, Nahid, as she faced uterine cancer. Nahid's journey was a testament to the resilience and power embedded in the female spirit. Refusing to allow someone to define her process and her time frame, she chose understanding over fear, curiosity over despair, and joy over suffering. Dr. Darvish's vulnerability and strength as she shares her mother's journey and her own, carried on from previous generations, is showcased in the pages of this book, serving as a profound inspiration for women facing their own battles.

Nahid's journey and those stories that Dr. Darvish shares throughout, remind us of the importance of embracing self-discovery at various gates in our lives. She introduces us to the KHOSH Method™, a six-part approach that aligns with the holistic and cyclical nature of women's health. The method emphasizes the interconnectedness of physical, emotional, and spiritual wellbeing, steering away from the reductionistic approach that merely masks symptoms.

One of the notable strengths of this book is Dr. Darvish's emphasis on the individual – the N-of-1. It encourages women to recognize the uniqueness of their own journey, embracing the balance of science and intuition, and challenging dogmas that may limit their understanding of themselves.

Through the pages of *The Golden Gate*, Dr. Darvish seamlessly weaves reflection questions, sparking a profound journey of self-inquiry. The integration of biology and biography invites the readers to rewrite their own stories, understanding that the exploration of one's inner landscape is as crucial as comprehending the biological processes at play.

The book propounds the idea that symptoms are not merely disruptions but messages and messengers, urging women to decode the signals their bodies send. It reinforces the notion that our sisters, nieces, and daughters are watching – whether birth mothers, godmothers, adopted mothers, or doting aunts – the messages we impart to the next generation leave an indelible mark.

In a world obsessed with external appearances, Dr. Darvish challenges the prevailing narrative of the quest for non-attainable perfection. As someone intimately acquainted with end-of-life perspectives, I affirm that not a single patient has expressed a wish for physical attributes over the richness of life experiences and human connections.

The era of despair, that has led to a tsunami of suicides and opiate overdoses, marked by unrealistic standards and obsession with physical and lifestyle attributes, calls for a paradigm shift. Dr. Darvish advocates for the empowerment of authenticity, finding beauty within and without, self-love, acceptance, and worthiness. She frames women as daughters of God, vessels of life and creation, role models, and gateways – urging them to seek security within themselves rather than external validations.

I have witnessed the transformative power of adversity in women, be it through childbirth, chemotherapy, or various traumatic events. Dr. Darvish calls for women to surround themselves with supportive circles, emphasizing the oxytocin-releasing strength of such connections. There is a quote I have stumbled across, I believe by a woman called Cici B., that goes something like this: "Be the woman who fixes another woman's crown without telling the world it was crooked". Can you imagine? Imagine a world where women raise each other up rather than tear each other down!

The book recognizes the importance of healthy polarity and the interconnected dance of yin and yang, masculine and feminine, the concept of give and take, the equilibrium in the dance of relationships.

Dr. Darvish seamlessly integrates these concepts, emphasizing the importance of, as Dr. Bruce Lipton describes in his book, *the Honeymoon Effect*, which Dr. Darvish expands upon – to BE the noble gas, embodying equanimity in the give and the take process – standing on your own, filled with your own accolades.

The book delves into the realm of duality and the healthy interplay of energies, transcending the physical into the energetic. Nooshin's passion permeates the pages, igniting a transformative energy that radiates to all who encounter her work. As she aptly states, wisdom is reflected in the disease process, and this book is a testament to her profound understanding of the terrain of women's health.

The Golden Gate is not merely a superficial cosmetic enhancement of existing paradigms; it is a deep dive into the individual terrains of each woman. Dr. Darvish emphasizes the fundamental importance of understanding and assessing the unique landscape of every woman. It is a departure of the one-size-fits-all approaches and commitment to addressing the core issues rather than superficial symptoms.

The book highlights the mitochondria (near and dear to me!) as the true fountain of youth and elucidates the transformative impact of caring for and nurturing these cellular powerhouses. The call to action is clear – to embark on a journey that encompasses the physical, emotional, AND energetic aspects of our being.

I applaud Dr. Darvish for not shying away from the uncomfortable truths, backed by well-referenced statistics, challenging the prevailing medical system rooted in disease management. The obstacles to cure are intricately explored, urging individuals to evaluate the WHY before jumping into the HOW or WHAT of treatment.

Dr. Darvish echoes the sentiments of another wise friend and colleague, Dr. Mindy Pelz, on the critical importance of managing oxytocin, insulin, and cortisol, to address the root causes of hormonal imbalances. She also draws attention to the impact of toxins on our energy systems – physical, emotional and even geopathic.

Dr. Darvish introduces a terrain-centric approach, transcending the physical and embracing the holistic nature of wellbeing.

Her commitment to starting with the fundamentals rather than resorting to a prescription pad is commendable, signifying a departure from superficial solutions toward a profound understanding of individual terrains.

As we navigate the Golden Gates within ourselves, Dr. Darvish's book invites us to ponder not just the physical but the metaphysical aspects of our existence. It challenges us to be architects of our destinies, creators of our narratives, and stewards of the terrain that houses our essence.

In closing, *The Golden Gate: Unleash Your Feminine Powers to Graceful Aging* is more than a book, it is a guide, a beacon, and a clarion call for women to reclaim their power, embrace their authenticity, and lead others through the Golden Gates within. Dr. Darvish's passion, wisdom, and transformative energy echo through every page, inviting women to embark on a journey of self-discovery, empowerment, and holistic wellbeing.

May this book be a source of inspiration, illumination, and empowerment for all women who heed the call.

With profound respect and shared commitment to the journey within,

Nasha Winters, ND, FABNO
Executive Director of the Metabolic Terrain Institute of Health
Author: *"The Metabolic Approach to Cancer"* and *"Mistletoe and the Emerging Future of Integrative Oncology"*

"Happiness is a journey
not a destination."

Buddha

INTRODUCTION

A few years before my mother died, she and I were listening to a brilliant Persian-American comedian called Max Amini, who was joking about the ridiculousness of the patriarchal practices in Iran. From the moment a Persian man is born, his parents celebrate his prestigious status in Middle Eastern cultures by throwing the baby boy up in the air and calling him "Doodool Tala", or "Golden Penis".

His entitlement and superiority as a man is reinforced over and over again by his parents, family, friends and community as they celebrate his gilded and privileged existence in society by the fact that he has a "golden penis".

My clever mother, Nahid, was often quick to make a witty remark when comical situations presented themselves to her. As we listened to Amini's comedy sketch, my mom turned to me and said, "If they call boys "Doodool Tala, Golden Penis", then what should we call baby girls?" Shouldn't girls be celebrated too when they are born? After all, girls are the key to our future generations and deserve all the world has to offer them. After a pause, she exclaimed, "I know what to call them... "Dar Tala, or Golden Gates! Yes, that's it – a woman is a Dar Tala, a Golden Gate!"

I thought about it for a minute or two. Then I had my Aha! moment and said, "Mom, now that's a brilliant title for my book!" So it became official, the idea and title for my book were born. The Golden Gate woman symbolizes the power and capacity women have to transform our world, our future generations and our collective mindset towards a more just, more peaceful society. As Golden Gates we must understand, accept, practice and execute our womanly qualities and capacities to bring forth this Divinely destined new order.

We are currently living in an age of unparalleled growth and advancement, auspiciously named the "Century of Light". As my spiritual teacher, 'Abdu'l-Bahá, said: "Force is losing its dominance and mental alertness, intuition and the spiritual qualities of love and service, in which woman is strong, are gaining ascendancy. Hence, the new age will be an age less masculine and more permeated with the feminine ideals, or to speak more exactly, will be an age in which the masculine and feminine elements of civilization will be more evenly balanced[1]."

But most women have misunderstood our sacred mission on this earthly life, which is symbolized by the Roman goddess Venus, the emblem of the gems of love, beauty, feminine charm and sexuality hidden within each woman. Many of us have fallen into the trap of aspiring to a false ideal Venus. We think that if we place all our efforts on building our outer beauty, by surgically accentuating our boobs, reshaping our facial features, adding fillers to our buttocks, injecting Botox into our faces, getting tummy tucks, and becoming 'skinny girls' then we can achieve our true worth and recognition in society.

Yes, we may get recognized and become temporarily happy with our new Barbie doll figure and all the robotic procedural changes we make to our physical body, but perhaps it does not truly heal our deep pain and may not be in alignment with our deep yearning and meaningful purpose. We may not realize that as a result of our inner dissatisfaction, our sense of unworthiness, and constant striving for physical perfection, we are contributing to a declining societal mindset, one with a whole slew of disturbances that continue to manifest in mental, emotional and physical chronic illnesses.

Do we really understand the consequences of knowingly or unknowingly manifesting our deep sense of worthlessness and isolation for our children and future generations? What kind of legacy do we want to leave behind us as parents and for our community? What role do we want to play in the transformation of our future generations? How do we change our mindset, our thoughts and our reality?

I believe that Venus depicts the vital role all women must play in this day and age: to rise up to our duty to create unity in a world that is overly materialistic and in disarray, especially during these uncertain, post-pandemic times.

Factors such as increased access to social media, a stronger focus on physical perfection, readily accessible opioids and recreational drugs, overuse of electronic and cellular devices, quick-fix diets, procedures and mindsets, prescription drugs, toxic and unethical agricultural practices, and a soulless society lacking moral compass are making us individually and collectively, as local and global communities, sicker and sicker each year.

Cases of mental illness such as depression and anxiety, and chronic physical diseases like diabetes, obesity, autoimmune diseases and cancer continue to spiral, affecting more children and teenagers than ever before. As actor, comedian and philanthropist Rainn Wilson writes in his book *Soul Boom*, we urgently need a spiritual revolution to overcome the current mental health crisis. I would add, to overcome our complex physical health crisis too.

As an integrative naturopathic medical doctor, my mission has been, and continues to be, to address and provide solutions to America's growing chronic health crisis while working on ways to optimize each individual's longevity to maximize our time on this earth so we can achieve our meaningful purpose. In short, to transform lives from within.

For the 28-plus years I have been in practice, I am grateful for the opportunity I have been given each day to serve my patients by helping them heal from chronic diseases and emotional trauma while extending their longevity, optimizing their physical and mental function, and improving their quality of life. Ultimately, I work to be a vehicle of transformation, to create opportunities for and raise people's joy, health and happiness.

Throughout this book, I will share some of the tools and insights I have acquired through my life-long education as an integrative, regenerative naturopathic physician and an American-Canadian-Persian Baha'i woman. In addition to my 28 years of practice as a physician, I have had the privilege of being a mother of three girls for the past 26 years and married for over 30 years. My personal aim has been to become the best I can be physically, mentally, emotionally and spiritually while creating balance in my life and in my soul. This goal encourages me to work continually towards transforming myself into a woman who shows up with presence through each moment of life, one who lives to be of service to others, creates impactful relationships, and is a Golden Gate in the New World Order.

Designing the Golden Gate woman for the New Age is a complex process, requiring a systematic approach to the transformation of our mind, body and spirit. Through the lens of my own personal, medical and spiritual journey, I have created a six-step approach, called the KHOSH Method™ (the Joy Method), to help each one of us learn the tools needed to metamorphose into a Golden Gate woman, like a caterpillar becoming a butterfly. I have guided thousands of patients on the KHOSH Method™ with incredible success and am now sharing it with you.

All three sections of this book will show you how the mind, body and spirit are interconnected and dependent on one another. They must be brought into balance and optimized so you can operate on all levels at your very best, in alignment with your heart and soul and your higher purpose.

The first section, Virtue I, explores our mind and soul to provide food for thought, reflection, inspiration and understanding. Virtue II digs even deeper by exploring our physical being in more depth – looking at the science of our body's systems, such as the gut-brain connection, the microbiome, our hormones and our autonomic nervous system, to help you achieve a more youthful, balanced and vital mind and body using non-invasive methods that activate your own body's innate healing mechanisms. The third section provides practical plans of action, set out in the six steps of the KHOSH Method™. It is a roadmap that guides you to systematically incorporate spiritual matters (of the heart and soul) and material lifestyle, food and regenerative therapeutic practices into your daily life to optimize your physical, mental, emotional and spiritual health.

By adhering to the KHOSH Method™, I hope your physical and cellular health improves so your risks for aging and chronic diseases reduce, and your lifespan extends with vigor and vitality. Alongside these physical benefits, I also hope my method elevates your spirit to bring you joy, to satisfy your deeply rooted emotional needs, to improve your relationships with yourself, your families, your community and your environment, and to help you achieve your purpose in life so you can become a vibrant agent of change in a world that is desperately in need of transformation.

Becoming a Golden Gate takes time and hard work. Each step requires us to be present with who we are, trust where we are heading, and understand how we are affecting ourselves and others. We need to recognize our veiled inner beauty and potential as women, and then reveal that innate essence, a gift from God, to those around us, to inspire ourselves and others and steer us effortlessly towards an unimagined depth of transformation.

Our time on this earth is short and fleeting. But our duty is immense. By transforming yourself into a Golden Gate, we can unleash our feminine powers to age gracefully, while helping humanity advance to global oneness. Let us create a world where women can lead in complement to and collaboration with men and leave a lasting impact. Let us inspire and empower ourselves and others to reach our full potential and transform our planet by steering future generations towards a healthier, more peaceful society.

Together we must arise to our full feminine capacities to become extraordinary, authentic women leading soul-driven lives filled with purpose and joy.

Get ready to be happy and healthy and to achieve your destiny.

Get ready to become a Golden Gate.

Dr. Nooshin Khoshkhesal Darvish ND, ABAAHP

....

The KHOSH Method™ and any information contained
in this book is not to be substituted for any medical advice
for your particular condition.

Please consult your licensed physician or reach out to me at
https://drdarvish.com/
for personalized medical support during your health journey.

Remember the information presented in this book
is for educational purposes only.

....

Virtue 1

The Art of the Mind
and the Soul

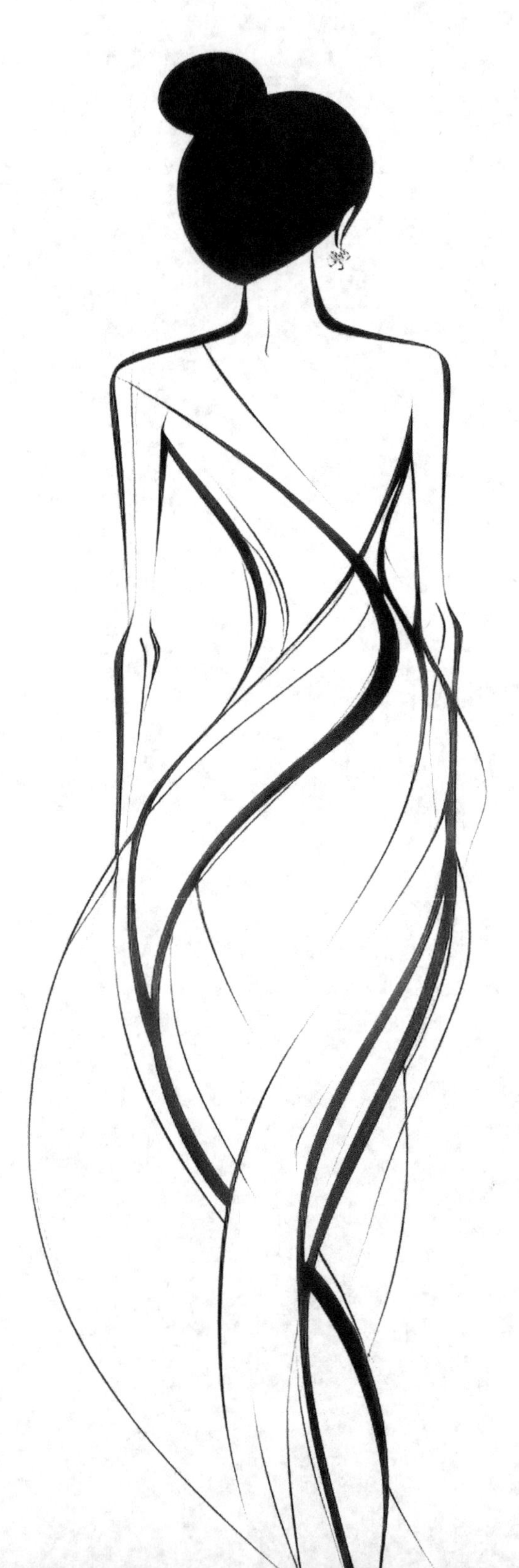

Chapter 1

The Journey of Being a Woman

"Yesterday I was clever, so I wanted to change the world. Today I am wise, so I am changing myself."

Rumi

I tell you, it is not easy journeying through this world as a woman. I know — I've been on this earth for more than 54 years.

From the day I was born in Tehran in 1969, I watched my mother attempt to fit herself into the cultural standards of being a woman in a patriarchal Iranian society, while figuring out how to rise above its prejudiced attitudes to women. Thankfully, my family fled Iran when I was a seven-year-old child and immigrated to Vancouver, Canada — only to experience gender inequality and inequity in a different way.

It didn't get easier when I moved to the United States as a 22-year-old Persian-Canadian female medical student. In 2002, the board of Overlake Hospital in Washington had unanimously agreed to select me as their first licensed naturopathic doctor on their campus. Before I signed the contract, I had a few questions for the three men who handed me the papers to sign. But each time I asked a question, the men turned to my husband, looked him in the eye and answered him. Not once did they look me in the eye to discuss a contract that I, not my husband, was about to sign.

I know I am not alone in this journey. Sadly, my experience of being treated as inferior to men will sound very familiar to my fellow women on a similar journey through life. To make our path harder still, throughout it all we have to cope with our physical changes. The monthly cycles of moodiness, weight gain, bloating and menstrual cramps last for an average of 40 years. Then there's the challenges of adjusting to a pregnant mind and body for nine months, followed by the intense laboring pains of birthing a baby.

Once the baby arrives, there's the challenge of sleepless nights and the painful nipples of breastfeeding – not to mention meeting the constant physical and emotional demands of a growing child.

When we think we are finally getting used to raising our children and settling back into the body we once knew, then menopause hits us and hot flashes, more mood swings, wrinkles and saggy skin become an unavoidable reality.

Of course, despite all these physical challenges, as women we also forge ahead to meet the day-to-day demands of housekeeping, cooking, cleaning and holding down a career. With a job description that may include mother and educator, wife or partner, professional, housekeeper, sister, friend, daughter, caregiver, business owner, student and employee, it just never seems to end. It's an impossible juggling act – and I hear you if you feel you can never meet everyone's expectations.

However, I'm here to remind you that alongside all the physical, mental, and emotional tests of being a woman, there are so many blessings that are showered upon us. The privilege of experiencing the profound concept of oneness through carrying and deeply connecting with another soul for nine months is the most precious gift many of us have been awarded. What a blessing it is to partner with another priceless soul from the beginning of its conception to the end of its time in the womb, and to have those magical moments of connection with our babies while breastfeeding.

And our monthly cycles, though troublesome for many, can give us an excuse to take a break from our mundane and frantic routines, letting us reflect, re-assess and work on transforming ourselves into a better version. Menopause brings more possibilities: to heal and recreate our relationships with spouses and partners as our children empty their nests, and to acknowledge the reality of our aging parents as we become their primary caregivers.

The challenges that cross our paths during life are purposefully created for us. They help us learn, grow and transform into a conscious spiritual being capable of helping the world move towards a more united civilization. What a precious gift we have been given: the gift of traveling through life on this earth in the creative, compassionate and beautiful form of a woman.

When we transform ourselves spiritually, we have the power to change the lives of those around us too. And when we cultivate a deeper relationship with ourselves and our loved ones, we gain a stronger sense of oneness, confidence and wellbeing. This helps us de-stress and improve our physical, emotional and mental wellbeing so we can feel youthful for longer and embrace the aging process gracefully.

My personal perimenopausal journey has been marked by many moments of elation combined with times of deep sorrow, anxiety, fear and grief. The darkest time came when my beloved mother, Nahid, was diagnosed aged 70 with an aggressive form of uterine cancer. Her oncologists gave her a maximum of one year to live – even less if she chose not to be treated with radiation and chemotherapy.

My mother, always a strong fearless woman and adamant in her faith, turned all conventional treatments down – including radiation and chemotherapy – because she believed it was the right mindful choice. Instead, she chose to go face to face with cancer – to understand the reason behind her cancer, to address the root causes of the disease, to use naturopathic therapies to support her innate healing capacity, and to make lifestyle choices that would help her become a more complete person. Even if she lived for only a few more months, she felt she would at least live a life filled with integrity, enjoying her children and grandchildren to the utmost instead of battling the side effects of therapies she did not agree with.

The Golden Gate Dr. Nooshin Khoshkhesal Darvish

Against all the odds, my mother continued to fight for nine years. Every time she went to her oncologist for a check-up, she was told she had an aggressive cancer and that she must do chemotherapy. Every time, she would come home depressed for a week or two. Then she would regain her bearings and fight with all her soul to prove to her doctors that there is more than one way to heal.

Instead of losing the battle to illness, for nine years my mother thrived. Not a single conventional doctor asked her what she was doing to look and feel so strong and well. No-one wondered why a so-called aggressive Stage 3 endometrial cancer had not progressed. No-one gave her or God credit that perhaps her time was not yet up and she still had a purpose to fulfil in the world. My mother continued to work as a real estate agent while traveling, visiting friends and family, joking and laughing. She set an example of strength, determination, faith and love for her children, grandchildren and community.

She also knew when enough was enough, when her destiny was calling her. In the middle of the pandemic in 2021, nine years after her initial diagnosis and one year after my father passed away, my mother began listening to her inner voice that told her it was time to be released from this world, and heaven was calling. The end came quickly. With dignity and respect for others, she called every single family member and friend around her and said her goodbyes while wishing each of us well. A few days later, on 16 March, she waited until her loved ones were surrounding her in prayer and love and took her final breath with a glistening smile on her face.

During those nine years of providing medical and emotional care for my mother, I began a new stage of perimenopause and then the pandemic hit. We became empty nesters when my youngest daughter left home for university. My husband and I moved away from the community we had called home for the last 16 years, in the midst of finding myself traveling between the US and Canada each week to care for my mother.

Back at my clinic in the meantime, many of my team moved away due to reasons relating to the pandemic. My husband and I were left to search for new people to hire while attempting to navigate the complex demands of that time: treating patients with chronic complex conditions, cancer and COVID-19 and processing the grief of the loss of my father and mother. Most people usually experience stress levels of two or three out of ten. At that point, mine had been dialed up to twelve.

I felt as though my life had been turned upside down overnight. Everything I knew to be normal was no longer the same. My body was not behaving normally, my environment had changed, my family dynamics had dramatically shifted. Everything had come to a standstill forcing me to re-evaluate, to reflect on my past, to heal, to grow, to learn and to figure out how to move forward in a world that was no longer familiar to me. I suddenly found myself at a crossroads, except one road was closed and I was forced to go down the other path with no idea where it was going to lead me.

So, menopause for me has been not only a transition from my fertile years but a shift in my essential relationships. I was forced to learn new ways of communicating with my parents in heaven, with my adult daughters who were no longer children, and with my husband too, as we navigated new ways of living together as empty-nesters. All these transitions unleashed feelings of grief and loss, of confusion and uncertainty.

Yet there was a quiet sense, too, of inner excitement waiting to take shape. It was the promise of opportunities for change, growth and renewal. I was given a choice: I could either look at my world as one that was falling apart, or one that I had a chance to recreate for the better.

My physical perimenopausal symptoms – such as heart palpitations, abdominal pain, itchy skin, fatigue, brain fog, hot flashes, weight gain and insomnia – forced me to stop and reflect. Menopause is an opportunity to look back, to be grateful, to heal unresolved emotions and traumas and then to close the book and open a new one. This new chapter gives us women a chance to act differently, to look deeply, to learn from our past and to reinvent ourselves for the better.

As I move through this life stage, I am constantly forced to examine my fears: all the sadness, grief, losses and confusion, plus the unresolved emotions that had been buried unknowingly during most of my childhood and adult years. The process of unraveling the reasons behind my emotions, the patterns I had repeated in my relationships with others and with myself, and the yearning to continue to strengthen my soul's journey during this period of my life, continues to teach me to be more resilient and patient than I had ever thought possible, and to learn lessons I never knew existed.

I started to reflect more deeply on some of the most spiritually enlightening thoughts and questions. As I start to understand the true meaning of love and relationships, glimpse the reality of our souls, and discover the generational reasons for our patterns of thought and behavior, I am learning to close the chapter of the first half of my life as a new chapter with exciting opportunities begins to unfold.

These powerful transitional opportunities during perimenopause and menopause help to further strengthen our spiritual qualities of patience, endurance, trust, faith and compassion. They allow us to become aware of our spirituality and the soulful qualities many of us may have forgotten since childhood. As we perfect our spiritual assets through the challenges set before us during the menopausal years, we understand how this wiser soul makes us able to cope with the challenges of our aging body.

This holds true for healing any other parts of you that might be needing your immediate attention. For some of you it may be a debilitating autoimmune disorder, complex illness, cancer, Long COVID, or another condition you may have. My menopause experience describes how we all can find ways to heal ourselves once we choose to live life with the anticipation of uncovering the infinite possibilities of expansion that await us – regardless of our current circumstances.

As you go through your individual journey too, I want you to appreciate that however hard your multiple challenges, especially being a woman, there is an opportunity to learn and to grow. You have the Golden Gate factor, and the power to transform your life as well as the lives of those around you. Remember, you are being forced to blossom into a strong, resilient and compassionate woman – and to develop and accept yourself as an authentically influential woman.

I use the word 'accept' because many women often fight the Golden Gate within by either rejecting or demeaning themselves, as they blindly follow the norms and beliefs of society and our family systems. You may have the unhelpful habit of listening to the quiet voice inside your head that is echoing the limiting beliefs that previous generations of women have been told.

The Golden Gate Dr. Nooshin Khoshkhesal Darvish

Perhaps you are resigned to this little voice because you may not believe that you, or women in general, can play a pivotal role in the advancement of society. Maybe you don't believe you have the capacity to change the world. Or perhaps you view yourself as small and have never really believed in yourself. You may not recognize that you are endowed with the complimentary, influential and noble attributes that are so necessary for the wellbeing and progress of your family, as well as the planet – or maybe you do.

Well, it's time to put all that aside and accept yourself as a woman who has the capacity and power to shift the world around you. You are powerful and full of capacity. You are meant to create, to transform, to grow. You deserve to be who you are in this world: a powerful authentic woman, a Golden Gate.

So how do we achieve this? As a woman, you already have the innate ability to be empathetic, to understand and to hear others. All you need to practice is to be present, to stay grounded and to let go of your inner ego – the one that may be saying you are always right, or perhaps you are always wrong or small. Or it may be the one that is telling you are powerless and alone. The possibility you need to entertain is that you are not always right or wrong. In fact, there is no right or wrong – and you are definitely not small, or powerless, or alone. Beyond the dual concept, there is a third dimension and we must all open our eyes, hearts and minds to it as we detach from our egos.

The challenge is to let go… and start to trust. As you do, you will find your gifts will manifest naturally. This is how you will cultivate deeper and more meaningful connections in your relationships with your loved ones, as well as in your communities.

Everything is about making mindful and empowering choices. Let me explain the difference between a decision and a choice. A decision is usually a masculine form of resolution. It is a conclusion a person makes after all options have been analyzed and evaluated, and it is made purely by thinking while ignoring the heart. A choice, on the other hand, is generally a feminine way of reaching a conclusion. It is a declaration from the heart about what makes the heart and soul happy. It is about trusting your intuition and listening to your inner voice.

Neither process is complete by itself, however. What we need is a process that fuses the best of the brain and the soul – what I call 'mindful choices'. Conclusions based on mindful choices are made by listening to the heart and intuition, while allowing the mind and brain to ground the soul. It is about balancing the wisdom of all parts of your being, the soul, heart and brain, to finalize a verdict.

For instance, making a medical judgment is not just about statistics and the science of medicine. It is about generating a balance between what science says and what intuition and the soul say about the condition of the patient. The combination provides the source for an individualized and personalized medicine. This type of medicine is far more comprehensive and effective at finding the root causes of disease and healing the patient than either method used alone.

It is all about balance. Consider mindfully choosing to rise to your duty as a woman, creating an alignment between your mind, body, soul and heart to lead society towards moderation. As you arise to your destiny as a Golden Gate, alongside every other woman, your strengths will start to balance those of men, and society will be able to accomplish its higher purpose as an ever-advancing, unified global society.

Arising to your station as a noble woman will not be easy. But the challenge of shifting society towards the ancient ideal of the goddess Venus will elevate your mind and soul and promote wellbeing. When you start to lead a fulfilling life your cells rejuvenate too, slowing the aging process and preserving your youthful appearance.

Reflection questions

- Think about where you are on your journey through life as a woman. What are the particular physical and emotional challenges you are facing? How can you use these to reflect on what you can do to learn and to grow, and to heal your unresolved emotional blocks from the past?

- My mother taught me to be graceful, kind and determined and to live with integrity, humor, truthfulness, authenticity and self-acceptance. Which women have helped you develop over your life, and which qualities and lessons have they taught you? Which men are a positive force in your life?

- Observe if the women around you run their lives based on choices, decisions or mindful choices. Do you mindfully choose to be comfortable in your own skin and practice your strengths as a woman? Or do you overlook your feminine qualities and function in a masculine manner, thinking it's the only way to success?

Thank you, men!

In your role as a woman, you may have forgotten that men play a pivotal role in shaping you into the woman you become. You may have bought into men's societal attitudes, stemming from the Middle Eastern culture of 'golden penis' and strengthened by Charles Darwin's evolutionary theory of the survival of the fittest, promoting the idea that women are intellectually and physically inferior to men. With each subsequent generation, the illusion of women as the weaker sex has been reinforced, and we now have the difficult task of correcting it.

But perhaps Darwin's inferiority theory hasn't been so great an obstacle to women's development as we think. I believe it has actually played a quiet yet powerful role in giving women inner strength, resilience and wisdom. Look at some of the women around you who have rebelled against this inferiority theory and risen to recognized positions in society. Oprah Winfrey, Michelle Obama and Hillary Clinton are examples of thousands who have shifted society's mindset by rebelling gracefully against the patriarchy.

The bottom line: while men challenge women, they also push women beyond our comfort zone, obliging us to grow in ways we never knew we had the capacity for. So, thank you men for helping women become more resilient and more powerful!

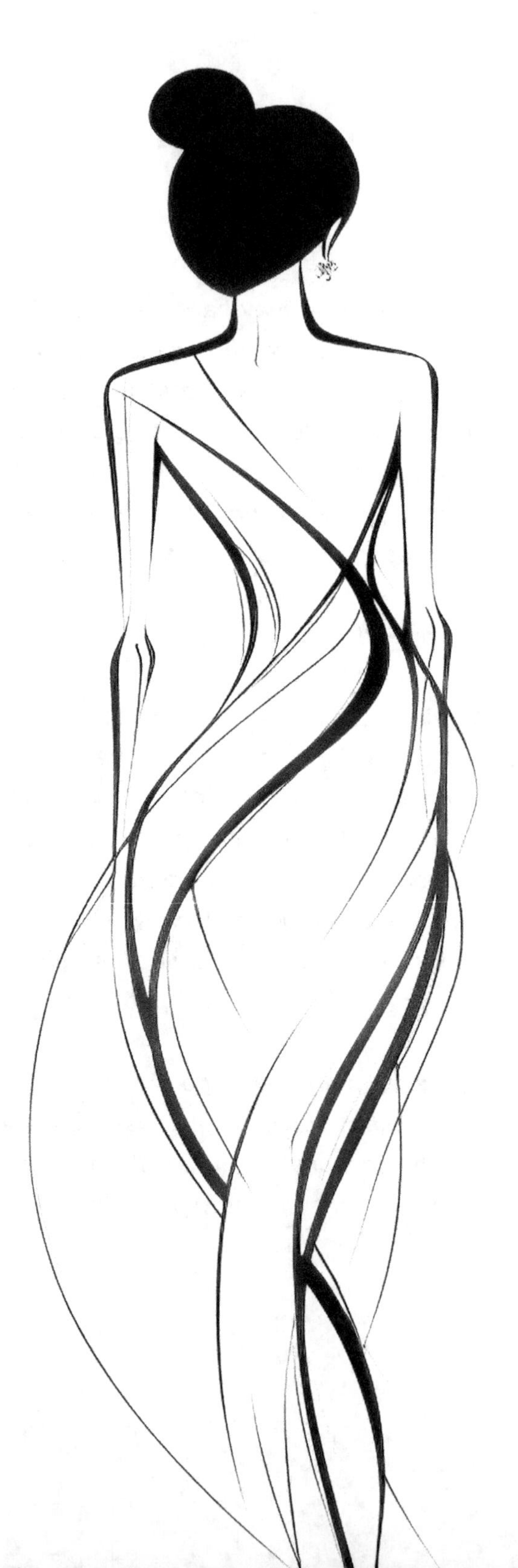

Chapter 2

Drama, Trauma and Victories

"The male and female
are like the two wings
of a bird and when both
wings are reinforced
with the same impulse
the bird of humanity
will be enabled to soar
heavenward to the summit
of progress."

'Abdu'l-Bahá

Women have been unjustly oppressed, discriminated against and attacked physically, emotionally and sexually for thousands of years. In many countries, even today, women continue to be treated as second-class citizens. They are frequently raped, violated, genitally mutilated and married off as young children. Inequalities in laws pertaining to marriage, marital wealth, divorce, and child custody still exist today[1]. In many countries, women are denied basic education and restricted to minimal human rights.

Women of the Middle East have been persecuted and abused and forced to wear clothing and covering that prohibits them from revealing their beautiful face and hair. They have been forbidden to pray in the same chamber as men, and have even been forced to live a lifetime under house arrest with no windows. Despite centuries of trying to make their voices heard, women across the globe are still struggling to be accepted as the equal of men – let alone being acknowledged as a complement to the patriarchy.

Today, in the West, some women fight to be seen as men's equals by denying their feminine gifts and acting as alpha males do, with aggression and dominating behavior, both at work and in their personal lives. At the other end of the spectrum, other women continue to feel small, vulnerable and unconfident, doubting themselves as effective and necessary components of society. Both approaches lead to unhappy lives, stress, inflammation, aging and genomic changes — ultimately providing a disservice to ourselves, our children, our families, communities, and future generations.

Let's recognize that women, as Barbara Davis (Zanotti) has said[2], "are the bearers of life-loving energy". She wrote: "Ours is the task of deepening that passion for life and separating from all that threatens life, all that diminishes life; becoming who we are as women; telling/

living the truth of our lives; shifting the weight of the world." As a female you have the power to be a leader at the forefront of society, taking the world out of a state of chaos and transforming it into one of expansiveness, peace and harmony through long-lasting solutions that will benefit our children as well as generations to come.

Every time I read the following quote from 'Abdu'l-Bahá[3], I gain hope about the outlook of future of women. 'Abdu'l-Bahá, son of Baha'u'llah, succinctly describes the role of women in this new age, this ever-advancing Century of Light. "The world in the past has been ruled by force, and man has dominated over women by reason of his more forceful and aggressive qualities both of body and mind.

"But the balance is already shifting. Force is losing its weight and mental alertness, intuition, and the spiritual qualities of love and service, in which woman is strong, are gaining ascendancy. Hence the new age will be an age less masculine, and more permeated with the feminine ideals or, to speak more exactly, [it] will be an age in which the masculine and feminine elements of civilization will be more evenly balanced."

Unified in our thoughts and approach, we must acknowledge and refine the gifts we have been given as women. Our capacity to love, our sensitive, intuitive, delicate nature and our ability to rise to spiritual heights are some of the virtues we must exercise in a world ruled by belligerence and displays of power.

Instead of struggling to become like men and practicing our masculine qualities, we must stay confident in our complementary womanly virtues and assets. Once these feminine strengths become aligned to complement that of the man's, balance in our world will be created, leading to the promotion and progress of a unified human society.

A Short History of the Women's Rights Movement

Elizabeth Cady Stanton, a young housewife and mother, turned to her four women friends at teatime in Upstate New York to share her frustrations with the limitations placed upon women under America's new democracy. That was 13 July 1848. That teatime marked the first women's rights movement meeting in the West, shifting the trajectory of women's rights in the US[4].

But the global women's rights movement did not begin in New York in July 1848. It was a month earlier in June 1848, in the East, in the city of Badasht in Persia, when a young woman by the name of Tahirih, meaning the "Pure One", ignited a spark that was to shift the world towards recognizing the importance of equal rights of women.

Because of her subordinate status in society, Tahirih – like other women of her time – only went out in public wearing a chador: a long veil that covered her from head to toe. Tahirih was the daughter of a prominent Muslim clergy, and was described by Shoghi Effendi, the Guardian of the Baha'i Faith, as a "fair and spotless emblem of chastity and the incarnation of the holy Fatimih"[5].

Tahirih made history when she decided to walk into a room where a group of men had gathered. With dignity, poise and confidence, she unveiled herself to the men as an act of spiritual modernization. The impact was immediate. Shoghi Effendi further writes[6]: "She, of such stainless purity, so reverenced that even to gaze at her shadow was deemed an improper act, appeared for a moment in the eyes of her scandalized beholders, to have defamed herself... Fear, anger and bewilderment swept their inmost souls and stunned their faculties."

Overcome by shock and deeply insulted by her action, many of these men could not bear the shame of witnessing such an event. In utter dismay, a few ended their own lives almost instantaneously. One slashed his throat with his own hand. Religious leaders and government officials were also scandalized by Tahirih's brave and unorthodox behavior. She was placed under house arrest for four years, then strangled and her body dumped in a well. Her final words were reported to be: "You can kill me as soon as you like, but you cannot stop the emancipation of women[7]."

Tahirih was a martyr whose courage, integrity and authenticity were exemplary. In a country such as Persia, now modern-day Iran, where women are still oppressed today, it is hard to imagine how she had the bravery to stand up for the sacred rights of women and her spiritual beliefs in the 19th century. She was the first woman in the history of Persia – and possibly the world – to stand up in public to show that women are equal to men, and she did so with elegance, beauty and refinement.

Tahirih was neither hostile nor docile. She simply displayed her feminine beauty and persona, exemplifying the greatest strength and capacity that a woman possesses. She is one woman who truly got what it meant to be a woman and lived her destiny to the utmost. Her story of influence, integrity, passion and purity is a story that all of us women should create in our own lives too. Through her life-loving passion and living her truth, she has undoubtedly forever shifted the weight of the world.

I strongly believe that Tahirih's act of unveiling was more potent than any man could have imagined. The energy released by her action was so powerful that a month later in 1848, the first meeting to address women's rights in the US, the Seneca Falls Convention, took place.

Tahirih's courageous protest triggered a ripple effect worldwide, unleashing a wave of women's rights movements throughout the United States, China, Europe and Australia that continues to light the world today.

In Fall 2022, the world celebrated the birth of "Women, Life, Freedom", the world's first revolutionary women's movement led by women and young girls in Iran. It was galvanized by a response to centuries of suffering from inequality, injustice, oppression and gender discrimination. Despite the activism that began with Tahirih in 1848, the atrocities, the injustices and the oppression of women continue, especially in Iran and the Middle Eastern countries. In the West, women may not be persecuted but many are still belittled and denied their inherent rights covertly. In the US today, many working women still earn less for the same position as a man, they are less likely to be selected to leadership status, and they are often denied respect.

The "Women, Life, Freedom" movement started in a small town in Iran after the barbaric treatment of Mahsa Jina Amini, a 22-year-old woman who died in police custody four days after being inhumanely punished by police for not fully covering her hair under her hijab. Since the start of worldwide protests against her death in September 2022, it is estimated that more than 20,000 people, both men and women, have been detained and imprisoned and more than 500 killed by Iran's Islamic regime for supporting the revolutionary women's movement[8]. Many are highly educated, including scholars, lawyers, journalists, doctors, and engineers.

Mahnaz Parakand, an Iranian lawyer and women's rights advocate, shared her thoughts in an interview on 29 November 2022 with the Office of the United Nations High Commissioner for Human Rights[9]. She said: "I felt discrimination in my flesh, skin and bones. I grew up in Tehran in a poor family, in a patriarchal community where socially and economically active girls and women were easily judged and rejected from society. My father, while being proud of my capabilities, did not want me to continue my studies at university, due to the fear of judgment from neighbors and other people around us. At the same time, he encouraged my older brother to continue his studies. Although my father did not stop me from pursuing a university education, I could see the look of disappointment in his eyes and this made me feel very upset and guilty.

"That is when I witnessed first-hand the inequality, discrimination and unfair judgment of society against women. I decided to start fighting for my human rights from within my own family, engaging with my father and brother to bring to their attention the unjust situation of women. My mother was always my supporter. In 1978, when I was admitted to the Faculty of Law of Tehran University, only 20 per cent of students were women."

At the age of 22, Mahnaz was arrested for taking part in political demonstrations and imprisoned alongside hundreds of other women. As soon as she entered prison she was tortured by being beaten all over her body with batons and gun butts. She was also struck on the soles of her feet with electric cables, which left her unable to walk or even wear shoes. The interrogation lasted three months.

Mahnaz reports[10]: "They tortured me the whole time. They took me to a 'judge' who didn't give me any opportunity to defend myself. He declared, "Your sentence is execution." I was tried and sentenced to death as quickly and as simply as that. There are many descriptions of this type of torture, but let me just say that it was so painful and unbearable that I was relieved when I heard the death sentence. I knew that my life would end with execution, but at least I was not going to be tortured anymore, and this gave me peace."

As painful as it is for us to read these stories of inhumane atrocities and the cruel treatments of women solely due to their God-given gender, it is more unjust, as well as inhumane, if we don't do something about such injustices.

As of March 2024, the Islamic regime in Iran continues to violently attack women in its efforts to silence them, as well as those who demand accountability for basic human rights violations. The regime has redefined and enforced new laws and policies that discriminate against women in relation to gender roles, marriage, inheritance, family life, child custody, and citizenship. In the spring of 2023, over 7,000 young schoolgirls were quietly poisoned with nitrogen gas in over 91 schools throughout 28 provinces, with hundreds hospitalized with respiratory distress, numbness in limbs, heart palpitations, headaches, nausea and vomiting[11].

Women are not allowed to play in certain sports such as gymnastics and swimming, nor outdoor recreational activities such as cycling or riding motorcycles[12]. Nevertheless, women such as the 2023 Nobel Peace Prize winner Narges Mohammadi, a scientist, journalist, and activist, continue to do their courageous work to shift society even while imprisoned.

Yet these inhumane actions and discriminatory attitudes towards women only make us stronger and more resilient. Women have suffered and have been oppressed since ancient times. Now, as it all comes to a peak, girls young and old throughout cultures across the world continue to gain power and presence. More girls than ever before are enrolling in universities to complete their higher education. Female literacy rates rose to an astounding 92% globally in 2020, up from 70% in 1975, according to World Bank data[13]. Women are becoming doctors, engineers, lawyers, journalists and politicians. They are being divinely summoned to leadership positions.

These young, educated women are preparing themselves for a global transformation that can only take place through the rise of women. What a gift they are giving themselves, and their future generations. If one young woman – like Mahsa Amini, or Mahnaz Parakand or Tahirih – can achieve such a positive global impact on their own, imagine the impact that millions of young women across the globe could make on our future as they become educated. I hope I'm still alive to witness this global transformation.

Female Education: The Cornerstone of Health and Wellbeing

Let's face it: throughout cultural and religious history, girls have never been the priority for education and they have definitely not been the chosen one in the family to be trained in the arts and the sciences. If a family only had the means to educate one child, traditionally they would choose the son. The daughter often stayed at home to help keep house, or was married off by the age of ten. Even today, girls in cultures such as India are sold off to be married at a young age while their brothers receive an education. But times are changing.

Let's remember that humans "are a mine rich in gems of inestimable value"[14]. An education that teaches a child excellence in character, high resolve, and awareness and love of fellow humans can reveal its treasures. Mothers are the first educators of children. If mothers are uneducated, we risk raising children who have little motivation to become effective members of society. To establish a progressive society, we must educate women so they can provide a foundational education for their sons and daughters. This education creates a basis for the moral decisions and mindful choices that men and women make, as together we create an upright, peaceful society.

I believe it's vital to invest in the education of women if we wish to usher in a new era of change and cause transformational ripple effects in our world. Educating female children must be given top priority. Because of my passionate belief that educating girls is critical to advancing society and alleviating most social ills, for the past few years I have served on the board of directors of the Mona Foundation, an organization that supports grassroots educational initiatives around the globe to educate and empower women and girls so they gain the tools to be effective members of their families and communities.

Through the Mona Foundation, I have met like-minded people with a passion to help transform the world by educating girls. Once educated, I have witnessed girls' virtuous qualities transform dysfunctional societies into ones that are strong and productive. For instance, when a girl in a small village of India is educated, she not only provides food and housing for her family, she also creates opportunities for others to use their strengths and talents to establish healthier communities.

I met Kali, a young woman living in a remote village of Alirajpur in Madhya Pradesh, in India in October 2019 when I visited her with a group of supporters from the Mona Foundation. Her story is one of empowerment and transformation resulting from education. Being born into a poor family in a remote village, an uneducated girl with a history of polio who had lost the use of her legs, Kali's future was dismal. In 2013, she enrolled in a six-month residential educational program for girls at Barli Institute in Indore, India, through a $350 scholarship provided by the Mona Foundation.

Initially Kali was shy and felt small and withdrawn. But then she began to learn and to find her voice. She learned to read and write, to farm organically, to cook with solar energy, to sew clothing, to run her own business and, most importantly, to improve her personal spiritual and social wellbeing and that of her community. After an intensive six months of learning, Kali – now more confident, enlightened, empowered and skilled – returned to her village to open a tailor's shop.

She earned sufficient funds to support her family and bought herself a scooter so she could get around. She became the first female in her village to purchase a property and built a home for all her family. She then built a second floor where she continues to teach physically challenged young girls to this day. Kali has inspired her community and other girls in her village to pursue education, to stand up for themselves, to become agents of social transformation. Today, she sponsors the education of eight girls from her village.

Educating girls empowers them to recognize their worth and their vital contribution to their communities, and prevents them from feeling inferior, powerless and weak. Teaching our girls and women about nutrition, disease prevention, hygiene, morals, ethics and mature mindful decision-making encourages positive shifts at grassroots levels in families and communities.

Educating girls to make elevated decisions, to raise their moral capacities, to be more confident in problem solving, to be skilled in the sciences and the arts, and to support their communities will create future generations that are physically, mentally, emotionally and spiritually healthier, happier, and enriched. Education is the cornerstone of wellbeing and health. Through education, human capacities are realized, lives are enriched and minds are empowered.

Women, Our Time is Here!

Ladies, we have sold ourselves short for too long. In a world currently dominated by alpha males, or "doodool talas", we have forgotten who we really are and have chosen to either behave like men in an aggressive dominant fashion, or convince ourselves that we are small, subordinate and powerless.

But the women's rights revolution that started with Tahirih's act of unveiling herself in 1848, and culminated in Amini being tortured to death in 2022, has created ripple effects that will reverberate for decades and centuries to come. In the year she died, Amini was included in Forbes magazine's list of the World's 100 Most Powerful Women. Nina Ansary, a historian and women's rights activist, has said: "Mahsa Amini is now a global symbol for freedom, not just in Iran.[15]"

Abigail S. Duniway, a 19th century women's rights advocate from Oregon, reminded us that: "The young women of today, free to study, to speak, to write, to choose their occupation, should remember that every inch of this freedom was bought for them at a great price. It is for them to show their gratitude by helping onward the reforms of their own times, by spreading the light of freedom and of truth still wider. The debt that each generation owes to the past must be paid to the future[16]."

Peaceful protests that continue to this day in every country from East to West are a testimony to the power of women to move the world. The time has now come for women to rise to be educated and to fulfil our potential. This is the next stage in the evolution of our human species, if we want to enjoy long healthy lives and to thrive. Without women, there is no life, no freedom and no civilization. Without women, there is no future. Our time is now. Let's seize the moment to fulfil our destiny and the destiny of humanity.

Reflection questions

- Reflect on the injustices and discrimination against women you have witnessed in society. Are you encouraging such injustices or are you speaking and living your truth as a woman? What steps will you make to shift yourself to live an empowering, joyful and authentic life?

- How do you think you can use the unique gifts you have been given as a woman to help transform our world to a more peaceful and balanced civilization, in tune with feminine ideals? How important is education to you? What steps are you willing to take to reverse oppression within yourself and your community?

- Try tuning into your inner voice as you scan your body. Are there any areas of discomfort or pain you have been neglecting or suppressing? What messages is your pain giving you? After listening to your inner compass, what do you sense could be the root cause of your pain? What guidance is your internal voice giving you to help you resolve the areas of pain or lead you to happiness?

Following *your* Inner Compass

Women have been gifted with an internal voice, an internal compass that guides us through chaos and pain. We can sense danger and recognize the presence of love.

A woman can sense when to be attached and when to let go, when to give and when to take, when to learn and when to teach, when to talk and when to listen. Accessing this divine gift requires practice, especially if you are not used to consciously paying attention to your inner voice. But once you learn to become aware of it, it will guide you to the most powerful ways of being and creating relationships and wellbeing.

It is all about listening to your inner compass and symptoms, then reflecting upon the messages your body is sending you. Practice this daily – make it a habit, like going to the gym. My suggestion is to set aside five minutes a day in the morning or at the end of your day. Take a few deep breaths, let go, and perform a total body scan. Become aware of the stressors or discomforts in your body. Place your hand upon the area of discomfort. Focus on it. Stay with this for a few minutes until it gives you a message, a color, a memory. Continue to stay with it until it shifts.

Your symptoms – whether a headache, nausea, joint pain, brain fog or fatigue – are your body's way of telling you something is out of balance. Symptoms act as a yellow light signaling "caution" or "beware". They direct you to look deeper within yourself.

Ignoring or suppressing the yellow light doesn't help you get to the root cause of your ailment nor resolve your condition. Often, the area of pain and dysfunction finds another outlet for its expression. For instance, headaches in your forehead may be triggered by suppressed anger or by your liver being overburdened by toxins.

A headache suppressed over and over again with pain meds may lead to liver inflammation over time. On the other hand, resolving the anger and/or removing the offending toxin along with hydration may improve your headaches for the long term.

Be patient with the process — there are no silver bullets. As you listen to your physical symptoms and gain the courage to look deep into your pain, the underlying processes causing chronic symptoms begin to be revealed. And as they are revealed, they often clear. A feeling of freedom and an increased sense of capacity then emerges. If you need an experienced professional to help you find and clear the hidden causative agents, feel free to reach out to me.

So be open to what your body and your internal compass are trying to tell you, instead of grabbing the quick fix. Remember, life is a healing journey!

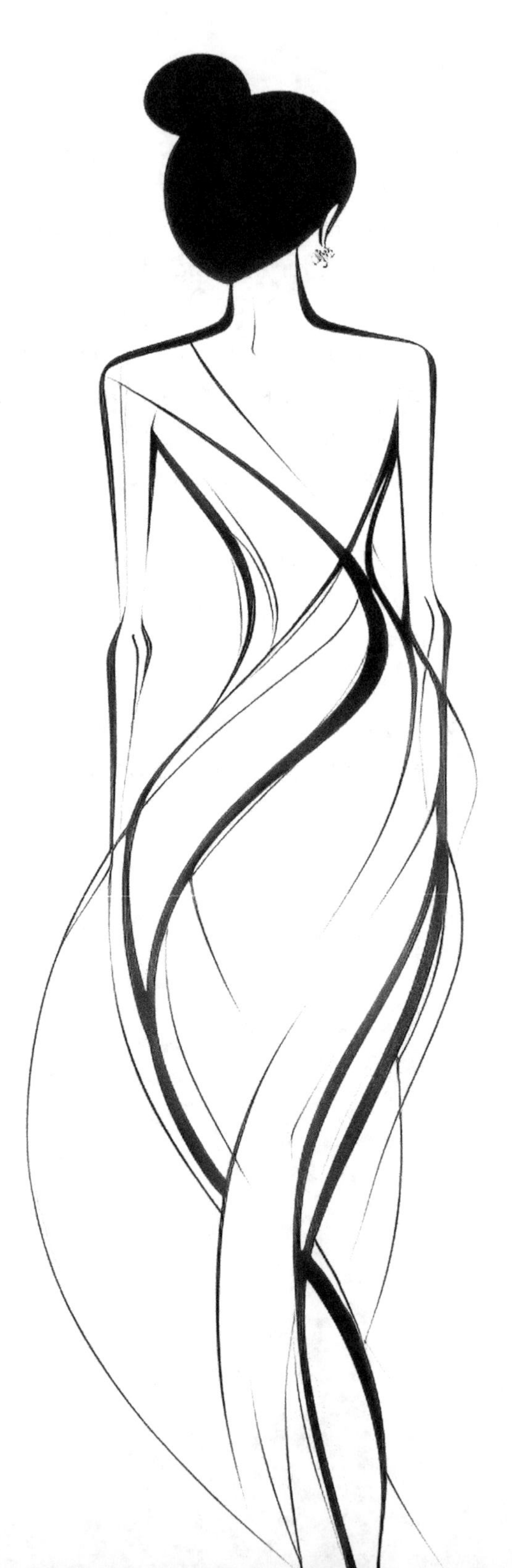

Chapter 3

The Beauty
of
Women

"The best and most
beautiful things
in the world cannot
be seen or even touched,
but must be felt
with the heart."

Helen Keller

Women have been the backbone of society for centuries. We are the Golden Gates that have birthed countless generations of thinkers, nurturers and leaders to advance our civilization. Without us, there is no future.

Despite our immense power, we still limit ourselves by buying into the idea that women are the weaker sex and that we need to look prettier to be acknowledged for our accomplishments. We need to go beyond skin-deep thoughts of exterior physical beauty and instinctively know that we are strong and powerful beings with the ability to make radical changes in our communities and workplaces. In order to empower ourselves, and to build a better future for the world, we will have to move beyond our current materialistic, superficial society.

During His 29-year ministry, Bahá'u'lláh, the Founder of the Bahá'í Faith, provided countless teachings on the advancement of modern-day civilization that can apply for generations to come. He wrote: "Abandon not the everlasting beauty for a beauty that must die, and set not your affections on this mortal world of dust." Whenever I become too attached to the material world, or experience loss or grief, or crave to change a body part that I feel does not look good enough, I use this quote to guide me to rise beyond the material world to an elevated, more spiritual space.

Feminine beauty is like a multilayered cake: beautifully decorated and delicious. When we set out to attract a partner, we accentuate the attributes that make us so captivating and alluring, enhancing our curvaceous physique, eyes, lips and legs with flattering clothes, fake eyelashes, lipstick and sexy shoes. Sometimes, we even get fillers in our lips and cheeks, facelifts, nose jobs, implants in our boobs and buttocks, and liposuction to remove excess fat. We put on a show for men because we believe they only see with their eyes and function with their little doodool talas, and not with their higher conscious brain.

But have you realized that by getting our lips puckered up and boobs popping out, we are bringing ourselves down to the level of men's basic physical needs, and forgetting who we really are? We stand in front of men with enlarged, jutting breasts, knowing that is what entices them. Then we complain they are not seeing us for who we really are. We are constantly reinforcing men to think with their lower conscious brain. What kind of a mindset is this, ladies? Friends, we are asking to be regarded as an object through the way we behave and present ourselves.

I'm not saying we should not accentuate our beauty, as looking healthy and groomed can lift our spirits and boost confidence. But by making physical beauty our primary focus and, in some cases, an addiction, we are asking society to look at us as stunning plastic sculptures void of depth, status and value. Just look around: we are starting to look like stiff Barbie dolls thanks to all the Botox and dermal fillers we use.

We spent $7.1 billion on Botox in 2022, a huge increase from our $1.3 billion spend in 2020, making Botox the highest non-surgical cosmetic procedure in the United States while feeding the alpha male Big Pharma industry. The Botox market is estimated to reach $18 billion by 2032[1]. In 2022, we had approximately 44 million elective cosmetic procedures in the USA. Of those, 244,000 procedures were performed on girls under the age of 19 and over 10 million were performed on women aged between 40 and 54[2]. In the same year, we spent over $8.5 billion on elective and cosmetic surgeries, and the numbers continue to grow exponentially for younger ages[3].

Yet we are not at all ashamed. Perhaps we have closed our eyes to the fact that our actions reinforce to our children the importance of physical beauty over inner beauty. We role-model achieving a perfect physique over the good manners, morals and spiritual virtues this world desperately needs so future generations can thrive. Then we wonder why the rates of suicide among our children and young people, aged between ten and 24, has risen by 62% over the last two decades[4]. We are our own worst enemy, enslaving ourselves to artificial methods that create an illusory aesthetic ideal while teaching our children to do the same.

The bottom line is that our fake breasts and wrinkle-free faces send a message of perfectionism and idealism to our daughters and sons. By reaching for a new false façade we hope to achieve confidence, yet we are hiding our true selves, our pain, our reality. With our new appearance, we may gain false and superficial confidence, but what we truly desire is self-love, self-assurance and self-respect. After all the surgeries and cosmetic 'tweakments', we still don't value or love ourselves. Sadly, our self-esteem and respect for our femininity has been lost.

There is a lot of work to do to help women look and feel authentically self-assured, happy and beautiful without Botox, boob jobs, or liposuction. I believe the healthier and purer our inner spirit and our inner physical body, the more beautiful our outer physical radiance and beauty. The more we work to rid ourselves of toxins and our deep-seeded pains, while aligning our soul with our purpose and nourishing our cells and soul, the more attractive, radiant and beautiful we become. So, let's look within ourselves and reflect on the reasons we may choose to indulge in elective cosmetic procedures — are they to numb our deep pain or distract us from our true mission?

The Golden Gate Dr. Nooshin Khoshkhesal Darvish

Women want security. We want to feel secure in our relationships, our careers, our family life, our finances and our futures. Isn't that why we get breast-lifts, facelifts, fillers and Botox? It's all about making sure we are accepted and secure in our relationships and in the world. We think if we have our boobs enlarged, our lips blown up and our wrinkles removed, we are portraying a more attractive woman whom every partner and employer would want to hold on to.

Well, I have a surprise for you ladies. Most men don't really want enormous boobs and they couldn't care less about puckered-up lips or a wrinkle-free face. Put simply, men prefer peace and authenticity. They prefer us to be happy and confident women. The happier we are, the happier they are. When the men in our lives see our joy and peace, they feel peaceful too. Their calm and grounding reaction in turn helps us feel safe and secure. We become happier, grounded, more confident, authentic and at peace as a result.

A recent study by the University of Minnesota on whether women's happiness comes at the expense of men – still sadly an issue in some societies – proved the aphorism that "a rising tide lifts all boats". The research, published in the Journal of Happiness Studies[5], said: "We broke our results out by gender groups to examine happiness levels among both men and women separately, and we found that gender equality significantly improves life outcomes for both gender groups, albeit slightly more so for women."

So, instead of looking at men to gain our security, we must be honest with ourselves and look deep within ourselves. We have to understand that it is not men, nor our external world, that brings us happiness and security — happiness comes from our connection with the spiritual realm. The more connected we are spiritually, the happier we become. Happiness leads to tranquility within us and with our surroundings.

Achieving this self-confidence does not always come easily. It starts with loving oneself and our Creator's spirit within us, as well as within others. I often repeat in my head a quote by Baha'u'llah speaking on behalf of our Creator: "Love Me that I may love thee. If thou lovest Me not, My love can in no wise reach thee."

For instance, in order to see that my husband loves me, I must love him, otherwise I may be blinded to his love. If I don't love my Creator, then I will not recognize His love for me. It is like being in a dark room with the curtains pulled closed. The sun continues to shine outside, but if I don't get up and open the curtains I will never feel its bountiful rays and receive its warmth and light.

When we do not love ourselves, we may not recognize love from others – for instance, our husbands, family or friends. We keep those curtains closed. As women, we are excellent at giving to others but often we don't know how to give to ourselves. We want others to receive our love but we are not willing to receive their love. Still, nurturers require nurturing in order to survive. Any successful relationship always demands an equal partnership between giving and receiving among the parties involved and that includes the relationship we have with ourselves.

As a nurturer, I am always having to remind myself consciously that it is necessary for me to receive. I tell you though, it has been very difficult for me to receive and accept love from others, especially from my parents. I had to consciously accept their love for me. It was a process of letting go — letting go of the concept of feeling that I don't deserve love and accepting the idea that I, too, deserve to be loved. I see this in many other women. Many do not feel they deserve to be loved; instead, they give without receiving. After years of giving without receiving, they may feel small, burnt out and alone. The result: depression, anxiety and burnout set in by the time menopause hits.

As a mother, I also often turn to my young adult daughters and school-aged girls to teach me lessons and remind me of the qualities I need to work on. Today's kids are very intelligent and have so much wisdom to share with us, as long as we keep our hearts and minds open and as long as we respect them and allow them to express themselves freely. Setting aside the hormone rollercoaster of the teenage years, these girls are so much more aware of the needs of our global society. Their uncorrupted intuition and purity of intention are exceptional, giving them the ability to recognize and know the truth that may not be apparent to us as adults. Youth can move the world.

One of the most important lessons a young girl taught me took place in the midst of the pandemic. A beautiful seven-year-old girl came to me with extensive hair loss one month after she had COVID-19. Her shining bald head only had a few thin strands of hair left. Her mother took her to a dermatologist, and left as she refused the prescription of cortisone injections and methotrexate, a chemotherapy drug, for her daughter's hair loss. Instead, she sought out regenerative naturopathic therapies.

The little girl also suffered from asthma and other allergies, although she appeared not to let any of her conditions bother her. She continued to be joyful, always smiling genuinely and giving me love and hugs every time I saw her. I worked with her by first using food as medicine by eliminating gluten, dairy, and food coloring to reduce gut inflammation, and providing her with more whole-food nutrition.

We then used homeopathic remedies for emotional clearing, nutritional supplements and microbiome supportive therapies to address her gut health, and peptide therapy to activate her hair follicles to grow hair. Within three months, she had a full head of thick hair and her asthma resolved. Her beautiful spirit, gentle and loving radiance and her grace continued to shine no matter whether she had a full head of hair or not.

Consider if all of us women were as carefree of our physical beauty and radiated that inner beauty no matter what, and with grace and joy, just like this little seven-year-old angel. How much more joyful, free and healthier would we be?

The grace that this young girl exhibited in the face of adversity proved to me again the true inner strength and resilience that young girls inherently own. Our strength does not come from people around us, and our beauty surely does not come from perfecting the exterior. A woman's exquisite beauty and radiance comes from the matchless faith, courage, detachment and love that each one of us possesses on the inside.

By tapping into our inner selves and reflecting and practicing our inherent virtuous attributes, women whether young or old have the potential to emit such vibrant beauty that no one can deny it. Most of us are attracted to that real everlasting intrinsic beauty and not to the superficial beauty that must ultimately disintegrate into mortal dust.

Ladies, the time has come for us to rise beyond our insecurities, our fears and the self-defeating beliefs we have internalized for so long. Having self-confidence, consciously incorporating positive self-talk, and visualizing ourselves as educators and role models to uplift ourselves, each other and our families can help us all achieve an upright and honorable character. Consciously creating joyfulness and peace within ourselves also promotes wellbeing within our relationships and our environment.

In essence, the challenge for women is to embrace our inner beauty and resist the temptation to use elective cosmetic treatments to achieve false aesthetic ideals, some of which create blank facial expressions that damage our self-esteem, alienate us from our true selves, impair our personal communication and set a false example for our children and future generations while contributing to our toxic load. Let's find self-compassion and self-love, and believe in our natural beauty and capacity. Let's create supportive environments for each other by leaning on and learning from our mothers, daughters, friends and communities, and recognize that we are stronger, more resilient and more stunning together.

Women have immense potential. It's time to break free from the shackles of society's illusory standards for beauty and embrace the goddesses we all have within us.

Reflection questions

- Have you considered having elective cosmetic procedures to change a part of your appearance you are unhappy with – or have you already had procedures such as fillers and Botox? Think about what led you to consider these treatments. Can you identify any external pressures or beliefs that may have informed your thinking?

- Think about the times when you have felt at your most happy, secure, peaceful and confident. What had happened at those points in your life, and who were the positive people who provided love and support? Did you find it easy to accept?

- What values would you like to pass on to your daughters, or to young girls in your circle of family and friends? How can you help them build self-confidence and self-love so they recognize that lasting beauty comes from within?

Surround Yourself with Supportive *Women*

I have been truly blessed with a group of remarkable women around me: my mother, my sister, my sisters-in-law, my aunts, my three daughters, my cousins, my colleagues, and my girlfriends.

I have a very special place in my heart for all of them as they have always supported me, nurtured me, taught me, and helped me bring myself to account each moment. Even without them realizing, they have encouraged me to reflect on my thought processes, to shift my actions accordingly and to up my game.

Recently, one of my 20-year-old patients went to a Taylor Swift concert where approximately 99.9% of the audience were girls and women. The day after the concert, she told me that being surrounded by all women made her feel safe and empowered. She loved the special feeling of being in the midst of thousands of women.

At Holistique (https://holistique.com), our regenerative naturopathic medical clinic, the majority of my team members are women. We all care deeply about the wellbeing of each other. I feel constant gratitude to be around such loving souls who sustain me every day. I share my respect, love, knowledge and appreciation with them; they in turn show me respect, care and devotion.

These women feed me, make me laugh, and provide me with a safe place to practice, to lead, to teach, to share and to just 'be'. We hug each other every day and feel safe to speak our truths and to share our innermost concerns. We have a rule at our clinic: anyone who gossips does not belong here, for backbiting creates disunity and encourages injustice.

This supportive environment makes us all feel safe and secure and means we all have the freedom and joy to give our patients the attention they need while being our authentic selves. Instead of wasting our time on superficial conflicts and unnecessary hurtful games, our energy is spent assisting others in the important task of healing.

We are empowered to create, to grow and to thrive in an environment of peace, love, and security. And as our patients heal, they naturally and unknowingly help us heal too.

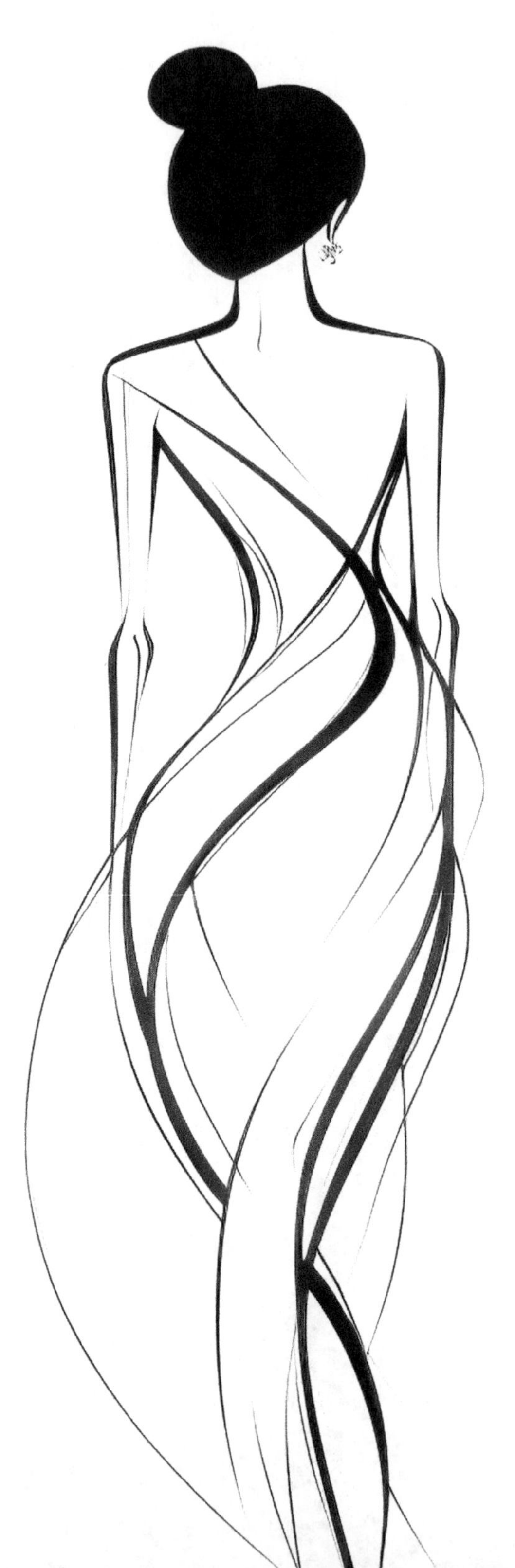

Chapter 4

The Dance of Duality

"The new age…
will be an age in which
the masculine
and feminine elements
of civilization will be
more evenly balanced."

ʻAbdu'l–Bahá

Men and women misunderstand each other frequently. The 1990s bestselling non-fiction book, *Men are from Mars, Women are from Venus*, by John Gray, sets out the psychological differences between men and women that create patterns of significant miscommunication and confusion between the two genders.

Scientists have been studying the differences between the brains of men and women for decades. They have been examining how the physical and anatomical variations between the sexes correlate to the differences in the way men and women behave, learn and communicate. I hope we can use this research to improve communication between the sexes to help unite us, and not reinforce our differences as a means to create separation.

I became more aware of these differences in the way men and women interact after I had children. As I observed the verbal and non-verbal exchanges between my husband and our daughters, I realized how a comment could be interpreted or misinterpreted in multiple ways by each gender.

Observing my patients' interactions with their family members also opened my eyes to how difficult relationships with those of the opposite sex can sometimes be, as each subconsciously communicates and misinterprets both verbal and non-verbal cues. My conclusion: the majority of us women don't understand or know how to communicate with men, and many men don't understand or know how to communicate with women.

Trapped in our own cobwebs of confusion, each gender perhaps believes they alone hold the truth. How conceited of us to think we're the only ones who know how to communicate, and that we are the only one who understands the other, while the other one is missing the whole ball game. We fail to recognize the multi-dimensionality of individuals' concepts, thoughts and emotions, and we may not try to understand others' perspectives by putting ourselves in their shoes – particularly when it comes to matters of the heart. Instead, we react based on our past learnt behaviors or trauma reactions. If only we were more conscious of the present moment and detached from our past experiences!

Hopefully, you have never been through a divorce, but many of us have watched family and friends go through this devastating process of misunderstandings and miscommunications. The anger, the resentment, the lack of listening, the pride, the disrespect for the other: these are only a few examples of ways we stray far from relating to the other individual. What are we doing wrong? Why can't we figure it out in a loving and peaceful manner? Why is it sometimes so difficult to create unity?

Our disturbed relationship patterns have reoccurred throughout thousands of generations, in every corner of the world. Most men and women agree that the fruit of the love between a man and a woman is children – because without children, humanity will not advance. But beyond this understanding, we sometimes get stuck. Many of us have failed to learn effective communication and listening skills to help each other's spiritual growth and development as parents, as couples, and as peacemakers of society.

We are trapped in our repetitive stories of feeling lonely and unappreciated. We are fixated on our weaknesses, our stories of being the victim, our unhealed sorrows and afflictions, our guilt and fears. We are attached to our sob stories as a way to protect ourselves from deep, unhealed pain. These stories have become our comfort blankets, preventing us from stepping outside our comfort zone and exploring new ways of being in relationships, so we can learn and lead fruitful lives of happiness.

Once we understand this, the steps we need to take to achieve happiness become clearer. We must accept and detach ourselves from our sob stories, guilt, shame and fears. Once we learn to be truthful to our inner selves, to respect ourselves and each other, to show compassion and empathy, and to align ourselves with the universal oneness, our communication and relationships evolve and become more satisfying and elevating.

When we trust our inner being, we are ultimately connecting and trusting the God within us and around us. We begin to understand that we are all the fingers of one hand, connected in ways we are unaware of, feeling others' pains and victories. We are all creations of the Creator. We become empathetic, compassionate, and full of love for others. We realize that once we express our thoughts and beliefs, they no longer belong to us.

They belong to the universe. In fact, nothing belongs to us. It all comes from, and goes back to, the Greater Universe. Our crisis and our victories belong to all. We begin to celebrate our oneness: the wisdom, beauty, and knowledge that each person brings to the conversation and the relationship. We begin to appreciate the ancient wisdom of duality, the yin and the yang.

The duality of human nature is well-rooted in the medicine of the Orient and the East. Yin and yang, hot and cold, sun and moon, light and darkness, and femininity and masculinity are only a few examples of the duality in our environment acknowledged by Eastern practices, including Unani, Oriental and Ayurvedic medicine. For instance, herbal medicines such as aloe vera, vegetables such as cucumbers, and fruit like watermelon are cold in nature and are prescribed to cool down feverish states.

Aloe is an effective remedy for burns as well as for inflammation of the intestines, both regarded as 'hot' conditions. Ginger and turmeric, both warming, are used to treat 'cold' conditions, such as irritable bowel syndrome and digestive weakness, as well as osteoarthritis. The Western world has begun to acknowledge this duality as aspects of Eastern culture migrate to Western society. Sweet and sour soup, yoga, Qigong and meditation exemplify some of the Eastern practices of duality that have found their way into North American culture.

Yet while we appreciate the duality of Eastern cultural practices, have we accepted the duality of the nature of men and women within ourselves? Yes, men, you have a female inside you and yes, women, you have a male inside you. Men have both testosterone (a male hormone) and the two female hormones: progesterone and estrogen. Women have progesterone, estrogen and testosterone hormones in different proportions to men.

Simply acknowledging the male and female hormones inside each one of us helps us become more aware of our similarities and oneness. Regardless of which gender we identify with, we are all part of the same humankind: like flowers of different colors, shapes and sizes growing in the same garden.

There are many more examples of duality in our physical bodies. In layman's terms, we all have both 'good' HDL cholesterol (High Density Lipoproteins) and 'bad' LDL cholesterol (Low Density Lipoproteins). Within our autonomic nervous system, the parasympathetic system (for calming, relaxing, digesting and healing) works in counterpart to the sympathetic system (for fight-and-flight). The female hormone estrogen functions opposite to the male hormone testosterone. Cells continually go through a process of dying off, and new ones regenerate.

The key to our bodies functioning successfully is the harmony between these polarities. It is like a seesaw: as one goes up, the other must come down until it's their turn to go back up again. In the middle they cross paths, understanding what it means to be up and what it means to be down. One gives as the other takes and then the roles reverse. Duality is all around and within each of us in perfect balance, oscillating from one polarity to the other in perfect rhythm and harmony.

One of our greatest challenges in life is to understand and be at peace with the masculinity and the femininity within ourselves, so we learn to comprehend and be empathetic towards the opposite gender. And as we attain more understanding, our love, acceptance and gratitude for the other gains more strength. Relationship communication becomes more effective and harmonized. We become more noble.

Becoming a Noble Gas

Dr. Bruce Lipton explains this in his book, *The Honeymoon Effect,* using the analogy of the periodic table. On the left of the periodic table are the elements that need to either give away or take a charge. They are givers or takers. Think about the chlorine atom, which prefers to take a charge, and the sodium atom, which tends to donate a charge. Together they make a stable couple – known as sodium chloride, or table salt.

A similar characteristic is found in humans: many of us are either givers or takers. Those of us who are takers often attract givers, and those who are givers often find completion when they pair up with a taker. At some point within the relationship, however, couples face the challenge of how to thrive and grow when the giver gets tired of giving, or the taker gets bored of taking. Either way, the relationship often falls apart.

On the right side of the periodic table are the elements known as the noble gases. These include radon, xenon, helium, neon, krypton and argon. I reflected on why we refer to these gases as noble. Noble gases have no need to give or take. Their powerful capacity is to be, to create, and to penetrate, diffusing their gases through space. Human beings' pursuit is to be like a noble gas: diffusing our essence of joy and love to the world around us.

When we become noble, we no longer need to give or take because we are mostly in the stable state of being and creating. In that state, we are elevated. We are strong. We are radiant. We are humble. We rise to act according to our noble mission. We then attract other noble gases with whom we can co-create a change in the world around us.

Our Biology of Beliefs

Exploring the power of beliefs on physical health further, psychiatrist Arthur Barsky states that a patient's expectations – their belief whether a drug or procedure works or has harmful side effects – play a crucial role in the outcome of their surgery. Positive beliefs have a life-affirming 'placebo' effect. Negative and disempowering beliefs can have the reverse effect, known as a 'nocebo'.

Orthopedic surgeon Dr. Ian Harris explores the evidence for whether surgery is unnecessary in his book: *Surgery: The Ultimate Placebo*.

A study from 2002[1] carried out a controlled trial on patients suffering from osteoarthritis of the knee. It found that the outcomes after arthroscopic lavage or arthroscopic débridement were no better than those after a placebo procedure. Dr. Harris also explores evidence noting that hysterectomies performed routinely on women for conditions like endometriosis, excessive bleeding and fibroids are unnecessary in the majority of cases because they provide no greater benefit than placebo surgeries.

According to the 2009 article published in the Indian Journal of Psychiatry: "Beliefs are basically the guiding principles of life that provide direction and meaning in life." It continues to explain that beliefs "are 'hot stuff' intertwined with our emotions (conscious or unconscious)." The biochemistry of our body stems from our awareness. Belief-reinforced awareness becomes our biochemistry[2].

"Each and every tiny cell in our body is perfectly and absolutely aware of our thoughts, feelings and, of course, our beliefs. There is a beautiful saying, 'Nobody grows old. When people stop growing, they become old.' If you believe you are fragile, the biochemistry of your body unquestionably obeys and manifests it. If you believe you are tough (irrespective of your weight and bone density), your body mirrors it. When you believe you are depressed… you stamp the raw data received through your sense organs… and physically become the 'interpretation' as you internalize it."[3]

A classic example is psychosocial dwarfism[4], a syndrome caused by deprivation, emotional stress, or neglect. Children who feel and believe they are unloved translate the perceived lack of love into depleted levels of growth hormone. The lack of growth hormone causes physical and psychological delays – delays which are reversible when the child is removed from the stressful environment[5].

Advancing towards this nobility is a spiritual process and requires conscious effort. To practice becoming a noble gas means bringing ourselves to account every day. It requires us to become aware of our beliefs, thoughts and actions and the impact they have on our health and the world around us. According to the quote by Russian playwright Anton Chekhov: "Man is what he believes." Sources of our beliefs may include what we were told as children, our environment, past experiences, cultural influences and religious teachings. Sathyanarayana Rao et al. in a 2009 study further explain[6]: "One of the biggest misconceptions people often harbor is that belief is a static, intellectual concept. Nothing can be farther from the truth! Beliefs are a choice. We have the power to choose our beliefs. Our beliefs become our reality."

We have the proactive ability to choose our beliefs, shift them, and replace them with new ones. When we shift our thoughts, we create new beliefs. And when we create new beliefs, we change our behavior. We can create new belief systems to pass onto future generations. Our beliefs strongly affect our day-to-day actions, our relationships, the way we perceive stress, and our capacity to manifest our health and wellbeing. This is borne out by a research[7] that showed: "Our interpretation of what we are seeing (experiencing) can literally alter our physiology. By subtly transforming the unknown (disease/disorder) into something known, named, tamed and explained, alarm reactions in the brain can be calmed down. All therapies have a hidden, symbolic value and influence on the psyche, besides the specific effect they may have on the body."

The impacts of our beliefs manifest in our physical health. Transforming our beliefs towards something that is more unifying, more noble, creates health within our body, within our cells. Transforming our beliefs takes conscious awareness of our thoughts and our bodies' responses to those thoughts. We must learn to become present and aware at every moment. This takes work. It requires us to turn inward to recognize the might, the power and the self-subsistence within us to overcome our challenges to create new beliefs and noble understandings. Reconstructing our beliefs using the nobility within us generates a stronger potential for us to arise to the destiny for which we were created.

A Beautiful Dance of Exchange

Becoming aware of our thoughts and beliefs is the first step to becoming a noble gas. This means recognizing that our thoughts and perceptions create our reality. When we think negatively about ourselves or others, when we think we are fat, or when we think we are powerless, we become all those things. That is what our reality becomes. And this leads to perceived stress in our cells that ultimately leads to disease.

However, when we think positive thoughts of kindness and love towards ourselves and others, when we think we have the capacity to change and to be agents of transformation in the world, that we are beautiful, noble beings, we become just that. Our positive thoughts help us become more confident, influence relationships for the better, and make an impact. Our thoughts regulate our behavior and our cellular health, which leads to outcomes conducive to our overall wellbeing.

Our connection to people around us is magnetic. When a family member is hurt, the rest of the family feels it. We feel the suffering of our neighbor. We are empathic creatures through the sole reason that we are united beyond the tangible. Our global society is falling into the depths of the black pit, marred by multiple wars, natural disasters, environmental tragedies, and epidemics of physical and psychiatric illnesses. As the suffering increases, some of us feel the pain manifesting strongly within our physical and psychological bodies. Our quest for solutions to heal this pain is becoming desperate.

So far, the solutions we have produced have led to a host of issues and detrimental side effects. We have not yet been ready or willing to listen to the medicine that has been sent to us. But if we bring the duality of femininity and masculinity within each of us into closer equilibrium and harmony, we will create a more progressive and unified human civilization arising from more tolerant, enlightened and perceptive communication between men and women.

Think about the wisdom of having duality in every aspect of human life. If it were not for cold temperatures, how would we appreciate the warmth? Without sorrow, how would we feel joy? If there were no wars, how would we value peace? How would we recognize friendliness without aggression? And if it were not for masculine attributes, how would we know to welcome the feminine qualities? Duality provides us with appreciation and motivation. Duality teaches us wisdom, nobility and strength. It implies the existence of more than one dimension and suggests possibilities in achieving our potential.

The moments when I have had my most gratifying communication with the opposite gender are when both he and I have been consciously aware of duality and have harmonized the two within ourselves before and during our conversation. Our communication becomes magical and fulfilling because each of us accepts the variance in the opposite gender qualities within ourselves and in each other.

We understand each other better. A safe haven is created, leading to successful and effective communication governed by empathy, love and detachment from our own thoughts and preconceptions.

Our connection is now more spiritual, more noble, resonating beyond the tangible. Our acceptance and harmony of our duality becomes the key to a beautiful dance of exchange.

Reflection questions

- When have you had your most fulfilling communications with a friend, family member or partner of the opposite sex? What made it so fulfilling? Did you consciously try to find common ground and see their point of view?

- Are you a 'giver' or a 'taker' in relationships? Think about how this pattern has shaped key relationships. How can you work on your inner equilibrium so you are either less needy or give less? What do you need to let go of in order to become a noble gas?

- What 'sob stories' of feeling victimized or under-appreciated do you often tell yourself as an adult? What virtues do you need to seek in order to let go of these limiting beliefs to improve your physical health and start believing in the rewarding and fulfilling future you want to create?

The Games We Play

How many of you ladies have played power games with your men? Because of our own self-doubts, fears and weaknesses, we try to control our men and force them to behave the way we want them to behave.

We sometimes coerce them to buy us the gift we want, give us the answer we want to hear, do what we want them to do, and show us the love and attention we want to feel.

Still thinking and behaving like six-year-old girls, we want these men to be our little Ken dolls so we can move their arms and legs the way we want. We keep them imprisoned and guarded in our dolls houses so they don't run away with a more beautiful and more intelligent Barbie doll. But little do we realize that we really don't have much control over our man or his behavior. If a man really wants to be elsewhere, he will leave sooner or later.

I have had too many male friends of mine share with me lately that their wives are detaining them in their own homes, like hostages. Their wives keep an eye on their every action, like a hawk. By controlling their every move, these women belittle these fellows, taking their rights away as husbands, as fathers and as men. Falsely, they assume that by controlling their spouse's behavior and actions, they will gain security and love in their marriages, or perhaps make themselves feel like they have power and status within their relationships.

These men play along with the game initially to keep the peace, but soon start feeling abused, victimized and disappointed. Desperate to find themselves as men again, many find the courage to break away from their wives to discover their freedom and true selves. Others continue to suffer in silence leading unhappy, unfulfilled lives.

We women attempt to control and discipline these men in a misguided quest for power. Then we wonder why we feel like their mothers as they behave like children instead of partners. These futile power play-offs only hurt our spouses, our relationships, our children and ultimately ourselves, leaving us lonely, vulnerable and depressed.

Such fruitless games hinder our progress and our health. They limit us from achieving our capacity as noble gases and arising to higher heights to be joyful and to create unity.

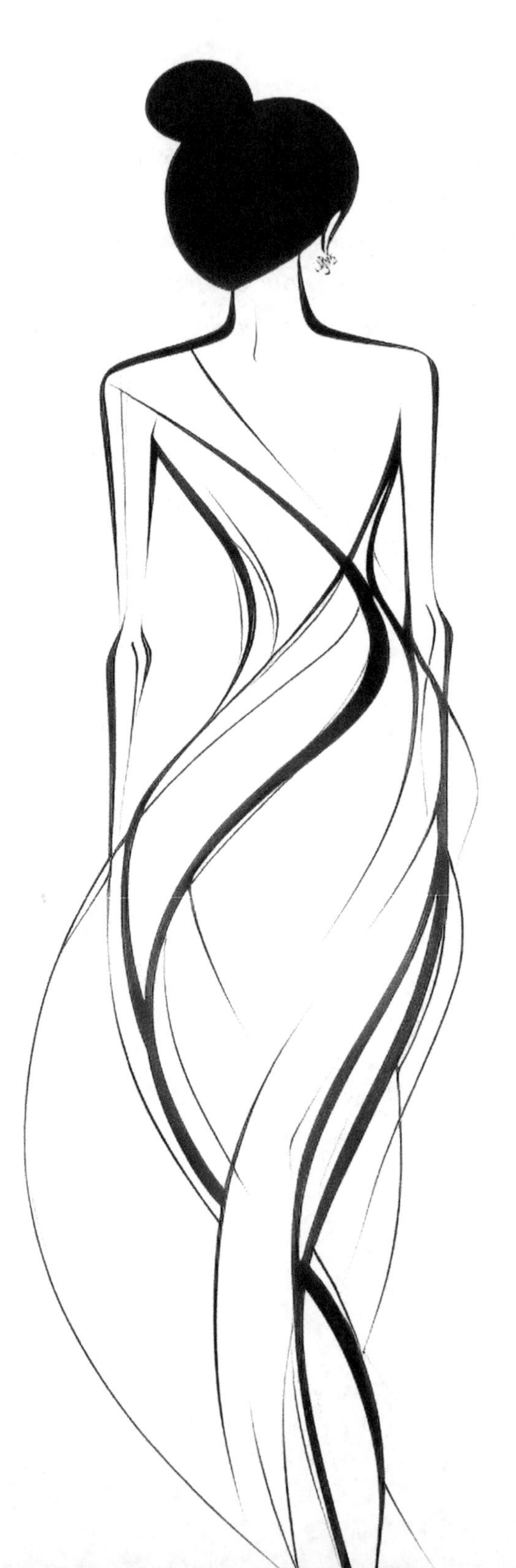

Chapter 5

Laughter is the Best Medicine

"*Joy gives us wings!
In times of joy our
strength is more vital,
our intellect keener and
our understanding less
clouded. We seem better
able to cope with the world
and to find our sphere
of usefulness.*"

'Abdu'l–Bahá

As I observed my mother during the final months of her life, it seemed she had lost her joy. I felt the depression she battled deep in my heart. I could sense the guilt she carried for surviving longer than my father, who had died unexpectedly a few months earlier.

In her mind, I thought, she was supposed to die before him. She was the one who had been diagnosed with cancer first. Why should she live longer than him? She felt alone without him, and her attachment to this belief made her health deteriorate dramatically. As depression took over her being, nothing could alter her mindset. She was determined to leave this world to meet my father again, and rid herself of the depression and guilt – at least that is what I thought.

She held on to life, however, to reduce her feelings of guilt at leaving her children and letting us down. It was only after my sister and I told her repeatedly that it was okay for her to let go and release herself from the fetters of this world that her beautiful soul finally freed itself from its physical cage and soared into the Realms on High.

How easy it is for us to feel guilt and shame. They are two of the deepest negative emotions that humans, especially women, carry within themselves – usually in silence. These deep-seated feelings of guilt that many of us have adopted are perhaps rooted in abuse and hardships we have suffered at an early age. Or perhaps our negative feelings are habits or beliefs learned from our family and culture and passed down through generations. We judge ourselves harshly when we fail to achieve the impossible standards of perfection we set ourselves. Guilt is our self-imposed punishment.

When we cannot achieve perfection, we may also blame someone else to shed responsibility for our failure, or we may react in an offensive manner – either by rebelling outwardly or by withdrawing inward, as a means of survival and self-protection.

We often find ourselves trapped by feelings of guilt, yet we find it difficult to pull out of this self-imprisonment because the burden of guilt we carry is often our identity. Without it, we feel we cannot survive. Guilt has become such a dominating partner that if we don't feel guilty in a situation, then we feel guilty for not feeling guilty.

Guilt is generally correlated to a sense of responsibility. We feel guilty if we have failed at our duty, if we have been dishonest, harmed others, or failed to self-regulate our behavior, such as breaking a diet or exercise routine. This inborn guilt and shame has become a blind spot for many of us. We feel guilty without realizing it. We often feel guilty when we experience a miscarriage, blaming ourselves for thinking we caused it by something we did, ate, or thought[1]. We become "bulimic shoppers" when we splurge on shopping and then return the items out of guilt or shame for spending too much. Some of us feel guilty when someone says "I love you", because we feel unworthy of being loved.

The problem affecting our health is that guilt is the most influential negative emotion affecting our physical bodies and our spirits. From observing and working with thousands of chronically ill patients, I have found that guilt is often the dominating emotion underlying most cancers and chronic diseases. These include chronic pain, chronic infections and debilitating chronic degenerative neurological diseases. A 2022 study found those who felt guilty were more likely to suffer with chronic disease, arthritis, low back pain, cardiovascular disease, asthma, depression and anxiety and even cancer[2].

Research on guilt reactions in cancer patients concluded: "Guilt is present in 93% of cancer patients and is responsible for patients delaying their pursuit for medical attention, for their sense of inferiority, inadequacy, and rejection, and for their inability to communicate.[3]" That research was conducted in 1953 and, from my experience, this concept still holds true today.

Guilt Weighs us Down

We can explain the influence that guilt has on our recovery from disease because guilt has a very negative valence. This is a chemistry term derived from Latin "valentia" that means "power" or "capacity". Negative valences often weaken the immune system leading to dysfunction of our cells. Once our cells are weak and dysfunctional, degenerative processes set in. Then chronic diseases such as cancer evolve and invade.

To make matters worse, guilt is often accompanied by a feeling of powerlessness. Our immune system is extremely susceptible to emotions, so once a person feels guilty and powerless in a situation, our immune system weakens, and we become unable to fight the invading disease. The weakened immune system provides a perfect breeding ground for cancer cells to thrive and multiply, and for a patient's tumor to grow.

From my experience of treating patients with cancer and chronic disease, those who have been able to overcome their guilt and sense of powerlessness often overcome their disease, including reversing cancer. But cancer patients have a significantly increased risk of death if they are depressed – and those who remain stuck in their negative feelings sadly find their disease progresses until they take their final breath.

The link between negative thinking and depression, anxiety, chronic worry and obsessive-compulsive disorder (OCD) is partially due to the way our brains are constructed and function, and partially due to the bidirectional connection of our brain to our gut, which I discuss in Chapter 11. Explained simply, the amygdala and hippocampus located within the limbic system in the center of the brain work together to respond to conscious and unconscious memories, emotions and threats. When the amygdala receives threatening information from our senses, it activates the fight, flight, and freeze response.

In prehistoric times, the fight, flight and freeze response ensured our survival when we were attacked by a predator. In the 21st century, stressors triggering our brain's emergency system tend to be related to cognitive stimuli, rather than to physical threats. Fears and worries about our children, our relationships, our finances and work, our health, our society, and our future can all activate our fight-and-flight response.

When we are stirred up by these thoughts, fears or physical threats, the activated amygdala signals for epinephrine and other stress hormones to be released from the adrenal glands. On release, these hormones increase circulation to organs and muscles, intensify the heart rate, increase breathing rates, and raise our blood pressure. In short, our brain tells our body to flee from danger. When perceived stress is chronically activating our fight-and-flight response, the tissues within our body begin to break down leading to aging, inflammation, chronic degenerative diseases and cancer.

Since the COVID-19 pandemic, anxiety and severe mental health concerns among young adults and teenagers have increased exponentially as a result of the trauma, isolation, and disconnect we experienced individually and collectively. Those traumatic memories locked into the hippocampus activate the amygdala to respond when they think about, experience similar situations to, or hear the word COVID-19. Such traumatic memories can set our hearts racing, disturb our sleep, fog up our brain, and make us anxious.

Approximately 45% of COVID-19 survivors suffer from Long COVID symptoms[4], as the trauma from the pandemic continues to plague our memories, immune system, and nervous system. It makes us question whether Long COVID is the result of the psychological stressors from, or the inflammatory and immunological response to, the actual COVID spike proteins and other toxins. Or perhaps both? We still have much to learn to fully understand how physical toxins, infectious stressors, and psychological, emotional and mental trauma combined affect our long-term health.

Negative thinking can become a lifetime habit if we are not consciously aware of the low frequency thought patterns we often carry. After carrying guilt within ourselves for decades, we begin to feel sick. We gain weight. We feel tired and lethargic. We feel depressed and cannot get ourselves out of bed. Our physical and emotional dysfunction now begins rippling outward throughout every cell to even our children and families, and generations forward. Our guilt is a hindrance to our progress.

To make matters worse, we seem to excel at magnifying negativity over time. It becomes a ritualized reassurance. We think of all the negative scenarios that can possibly occur, and then all the ways we wouldn't survive them. Such negative thought patterns stimulate a constant fight-and-flight response that leads to chronic symptoms, inflammation, heart disease, diabetes, autoimmune disorders and, ultimately, cancer in some people.

However, we have the capacity to replace these negative thought patterns with positive, healing emotions like courage, joy and hope. If we want to live the best version of ourselves, we must learn to make ourselves consciously aware of our negative thought patterns and then replace them with positive ones. By doing so, we free our soul, spirit and bodies from the heavy burdens of inflammation and degeneration, encouraging it to arise beyond the material world to perform its joyful soulful work.

During my mother's last days, I could see the negative thoughts she had fought against during her previous months were being replaced with periods of joy. As she approached the end of her time on this earthly world and was transitioning to the spiritual Kingdom, her mannerism transformed. She became more joyful, even though her physical state continued to weaken. It was as if her soul had attained its ultimate destiny in a joyful space. She exhibited so much joy that as she took her final breath she smiled a big smile, showing off her beautiful glistening white teeth. She was happy. It made me happy.

We need to understand that our attachment to guilt, shame and negative emotions are mostly rooted in our thoughts and bonds related to this physical world. When guilt dominates, our lower nature leads. In our higher nature, our spiritual nature, only joy and love exist – there is no room for guilt. When we act and work from an elevated place of passion, genuine love and joy, we are more likely to be successful at anything we pursue – we can enjoy a thriving career while raising a functional family and contributing to an advancing society.

Have you noticed how you feel and function when you go to work with passion and love rather than out of guilt, shame and stress? What about when you perform house chores from a place of love for the family? Or, if you are single, out of love for your own wellbeing?

Have you experienced how much happier and at peace you feel when you pray or meditate because you are in love with being in a spiritual state and connecting to a Higher Realm?

Passion is Energy

Talkshow host and actress Oprah Winfrey is a great example of how she has led her life by practicing all that brings her joy and excitement. She said: "Passion is energy. Feel the power that comes from focusing on what excites you." When we operate based on love and passion, an intoxicating glow inadvertently radiates from our inner core. Those who enter the electromagnetic field of such radiant souls feel the elation and are positively affected.

Serving others through love stimulates our own metabolism, health, mind and spirit while enhancing the spirits and health of others. Our minds become sharper, our intellect more acute and our passion more intense. The power of love and joy galvanizes us. Our eating habits become healthier, as do our exercise and meditation practices. We feel empowered as women and, most of all, as humans. The power of love, and not that of fear, anger, jealousy or worry, becomes our guiding light to transformation.

On a practical level, it is not always easy to replace habitual negative thoughts and emotions with positive thoughts and beneficial emotions. Sometimes, it is wise to seek out professionals to guide us and teach us tools to learn to reprogram our thinking, our behaviors, and our subconscious. But the benefits can be transformative and long-lasting. In contrast to guilt, joy and enlightenment have the highest frequencies of our emotions, and are regarded as the most positive for creating good health and reversing chronic pain, cancer and neurological disease. Joy brings physiological and psychological health and happiness[5].

Laughter has been studied for over 30 years as a possible medical therapy and yet physicians rarely practice it themselves. We hardly ever see doctors laugh with their patients. Our cultural beliefs have taught our intellectuals and doctors to be serious, because this signifies they are knowledgeable and professional. Yet, the best doctors that bring healing to patients are those who laugh with their patients, creating an environment of joy and positive energy.

Laughter has physiological and psychological effects. Stress hormones such as cortisol, epinephrine and norepinephrine reduce when we laugh. Muscle relaxation increases with laughter. A study on 60 women showed that laughter yoga – laughing while incorporating yoga breathing – has the same physiological and psychological effects as exercise[6]. Many physicians often prescribe 30 minutes of exercise per day but does any one doctor you know prescribe 30 minutes of laughing as a form of health prevention?

When there is laughter, there is no depression or anxiety. It seems that both cannot co-exist at the same time. So, if you have a friend or family member who is depressed or anxious, make them laugh. The healing that occurs for them and for you may just be something you both need.

My husband, Johnny, and my daughter, Delbar, both have a unique gift of shifting negative energies to positive ones. When they see someone sad, they first empathize with that individual, then intentionally create joy by genuine heartfelt laughter. Within moments, everyone including the depressed individual is laughing without reason. Joy and positive energy can be created into reality and are contagious.

At our clinic, we performed an experiment using a tissue oxygen meter on some of our chronic disease patients, including those with cancer, congestive heart disease and neurological diseases. A tissue oxygen meter measures the amount of partial oxygen (pO2) in millimeters per mercury (mmHg) in the tissues of the organ we are measuring. This measurement is different from the blood oxygen saturation level – the finger measurement the nurse uses to get your vitals – which measures the oxygen in the circulation.

We found that when we make patients laugh and bring happiness to their hearts, their tissue oxygen levels increase by 10-15 mmHg consistently.

It is no wonder laughter is the best medicine.

Reflection questions

- Think about when you last felt guilty. Are you aware of the hidden guilt or shame you may be carrying? If so, where in your body do you carry it? Do you suppress it into physical pain or do you project it onto other people, for instance by blaming others?

- How and in what ways have these guilty thoughts, behavior or habitual patterns affected your health, your relationships with friends and family and your career? Are you willing to practice joy and laughter daily until it becomes a new habit?

- If you are attached to guilt and other negative emotions, are you ready to let go of the deep-seeded emotion and replace it with healing positive thoughts and emotions like gratitude, enlightenment, joy and love? What support will you need to re-pattern your negative emotions and create a healthier life of your choice?

The Power of resilience

Resilience is an innate quality that allows us to bounce back from difficult times. It is a dynamic process that allows us to overcome stress and adversity while maintaining normal psychological and physical functioning.

Research has shown that women are more likely to experience perceived stress than men[7]. But the good news is that women have shown time and again that they possess resiliency in spades. Our resiliency helps us problem-solve when we face challenges in life. Perimenopausal women who have higher resilience as measured by their core resilience, spirituality, control, optimism, emotion and self-related resilience tend to cope significantly better with menopause, have less perceived stress and milder physical symptoms, while enjoying a better quality of life and wellbeing[8].

Studies have shown that resilient people often possess a moral compass or an internal belief system guiding their values and ethics[9,10]. Research conducted on 121 outpatients diagnosed with depression and/or an anxiety disorder showed that while a lack of purpose in life and infrequent physical exercise correlated to low resilience, the leading predictor of low resilience was low spirituality[11]. Purpose and meaning in life were key factors linked to resilience in a separate study of 1,081 patients[12].

To see ourselves in the light of nobility and strength, we need to have this inner compass, an unbreakable resilience that we all innately possess. However, we tend to chain ourselves to limiting beliefs that hold us back from the luminous opportunities for success and wellbeing. We tend to people-please at every turn and sacrifice our noble souls to an outworn, empty materialistic shell that the physical world has fed us for generations.

Expanding our nobility means having a growth mindset, understanding that women's innate resilience is not a static concept. It involves looking at obstacles as a challenge that can be overcome. We need to find solutions to problems by using our wisdom, our compassion and our feminine spiritual qualities, rather than falling into the abyss mindset of "I can't".

Once we understand that resilience is a dynamic process that takes us on a physical, emotional and spiritual journey, we can reframe our mindsets towards healing and growth.

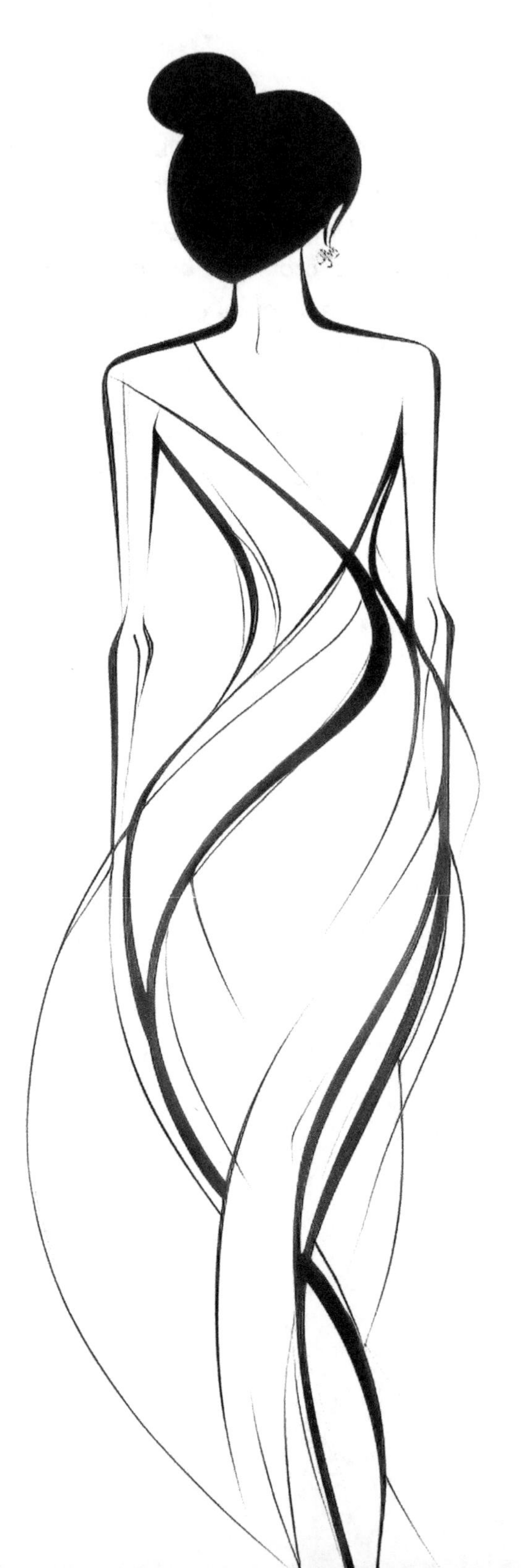

Chapter 6

The Wisdom
of
Healing

"To everything there
is a season, and a time for
every purpose under the
sun. A time to be born,
and a time to die, a time
to weep and a time to
laugh; a time to keep silent
and a time to speak."

'Abdu'l-Bahá

In February 2004, a patient with stage 4 ovarian cancer, meaning the cancer had spread from her ovaries to other parts of her body, was brought to me by her husband, son and daughter.

For five years, they had traveled the world looking for healing – from Mexico to Europe to different parts of the United States. For five years this lady had suffered, and now she was nearing the end of her life. She had been given days to live, and I was her final resource for healing.

After visiting her in private, she finally confided to me that she did not want to live and did not want to try to survive anymore. She did not want to take any medications, supplements, or undertake any new types of treatment modalities. She wanted to leave this world but she had been holding on for years for the sake of her family.

Sacrificing her own desires, she continued to dig deep into her physical reserves to travel the world to find physical healing only to make her children and husband happy. She was not able to face them to tell them she did not want to continue pursuing physical healing because she feared the truth would be devastating to her family.

After working with her for a couple of weeks, she finally gained the courage to disclose her true desire to her family – to be freed from the fetters of this worldly life. A few hours after she released her mental and emotional burden, her soul released itself from its mortal cage and flew freely to the world beyond. This was the true healing she needed: to trust and be true to herself and her family. She finally revealed her courage. As difficult as the process had been, she was relieved, as was her soul and her family. This was her healing.

In contrast, another patient with stage 4 ovarian cancer was carried into my office listless, cachexic (meaning with severe loss of muscle and body fat) and floppy in the arms of her husband in October 2003. Having been given only two weeks to live, her greatest desire was to live long enough to celebrate one more Thanksgiving with her family.

Her healing took a different form from that of the previous patient. After supporting her with homeopathy, adjunctive cancer therapies, nutrition, detoxification and emotional work, she gained weight and strength. Her tumors reduced, giving her an opportunity to celebrate Thanksgiving not only once, but multiple times. Physically, mentally and emotionally, she transformed into an individual with vigor and traveled the world with her husband one year later. That was the healing she and her husband needed.

Healing is an internal process far more profound than that which may initially be visible. It is a journey taking us deep into correcting the processes within ourselves. Biochemically, physiologically and anatomically, we may need to be rebooted and rebalanced. We must be willing to reconstruct our emotions, thoughts and beliefs to align with our soul's journey. This healing journey requires us to dig into the depths of our multifaceted beings to discover that which we have always known to exist, and to release ourselves from the bondage that has kept us ill. True healing takes hard work. We must find the courage within ourselves to move beyond our comfortable envelope into the growth zone, the healing zone.

The goal at my practice, Holistique, is to help heal my patients fully and not just suppress their symptoms through prescription drugs – which often leads to deeper disease processes that sprout up later in the forms of chronic disease, cancer and neurological diseases. When patients initially come to see me, I remind them that we are not looking to find a "cure" per the conventional model of medicine. Instead, we are aiming for true healing, through rebalancing the imbalances, eliminating the root causes of disease, giving the body the tools it needs to heal, and unblocking the pathways to regain full physical, mental, emotional, social and spiritual health.

I remind my patients that ultimate healing comes from a Source beyond any one of us. I, like many other physicians, am only a hollow reed allowing the Divine Wisdom in conjunction with scientific knowledge, nature and spirituality to flow through me to the patient so healing can take place. I also remind my patients that true healing may not occur in the ways we may want it to occur. Healing will happen in the form, time and manner in which it is meant to happen. We may think we need to heal at one level, whereas true healing may need to occur at another level. The key is to trust the process and be present with it.

When we learn to trust, our self-induced perceived stress response is automatically lifted. Becoming detached from our own preconceptions, power struggles and ego helps us gain peace with ourselves at work, at home, and in our relationships. This beautiful quote by American author Ben Hoff sums up the letting go process, detachment and trusting in a poetic manner. "The clouds above us join and separate, the breeze in the courtyard leaves and returns. Life is like that, so why not relax? Who can stop us from celebrating?"

Learning to trust takes a lot of patience. Patience with the situation, with others, with ourselves, with time, and with the Creator. It has been an arduous process for me to achieve this level of understanding and to practice it authentically. I am tested and challenged every day. And it is all worth it. As I learn to completely trust, have faith, and be patient and submissive to His will, I realize my need for worry dissipates, and I begin to feel at peace.

The Golden Gate Dr. Nooshin Khoshkhesal Darvish

People, situations, and my thoughts become a means for me to learn to be peaceful and to let go because I realize I am not the one in control – God is. There is no longer any need for scheming games because I know the best for me is determined by One greater than me. I trust that He is taking care of me, my family, my friends, my community and my patients. He always has, so why would He stop now? I remind myself daily of this process of learning to trust, to be patient and to be grateful by saying "God is the Most Glorious" (Alláh-u-Abhá in Arabic) 95 times. It is a process: a habit that is learned until it becomes intrinsic.

In an article published by Psychology Today[1], psychotherapist and author Dr. Ilene S. Cohen describes how trusting the process and enjoying the journey allows your joy to expand exponentially. This is about trusting your station and knowing that your value will be a determining factor in your fulfillment and happiness.

She writes: "You have to first be appreciative of who you are by creating a solid sense of self apart from external things, seeing your worth in the process of life instead of at the end of some goal. Some of us have gotten accustomed to looking at the bad and constantly complaining about our lives. That gives us the motivation to look for more, instead of seeing the value in what we already have, and it removes the option of being happy with our lives in the now. Most psychology theories teach us to look at pathology and what's going wrong in people's lives. It isn't surprising, therefore, that we often take on the same perspective for ourselves.

"In order to make a change, you have to train yourself to look at the unique, enjoyable moments you overlook as if they don't mean anything — like the fact that you're alive and breathing. You have to remember how special and fortunate you are. When you know this to be true, you'll want to experience life and enjoy the process. You're unique, and your life has meaning. No matter who you are, you have something to be grateful for; you have something to offer other than how many goals you reach. You have to believe that and honor yourself, your dreams, and who you are. You are a miracle. Time passes quickly, and you only have this one life to live; nothing is worth you wasting that."

Transforming Our Subconscious

Our built-in response to failure or to stressful situations is often to retract to protect ourselves, or to create subconscious mental or emotional blocks without realizing. These automatic responses almost always occur as a subconscious habit learned as an infant or a child. When an infant or child reaches out to its mother for comfort and no response or comfort is provided, for instance, those children often learn to withdraw inward to protect themselves. Over several months or years of feeling disconnected from the mother, these infants and children learn not to reach out for love and instead hurt themselves as adolescents[2].

Sometimes these children grow up to become adults who do not know how to show love to their children, or how to receive love from others. They develop a need to be acknowledged in the world, or to be seen and heard. When they find themselves in situations when they need help, many of these adults apologize for needing help or get frustrated that they are not seen or heard. They see themselves as small and unworthy of support or love.

They may spend the rest of their life looking for unconditional parental love. Sadly, they may not achieve their potential as adults as a result. They may feel like they have no backbone of love, or they may feel unworthy to stand up for themselves. I find these souls mature into bodies with weakened spines or with curved backs – we medically label this as osteoporosis, osteopenia or acquired scoliosis.

Osteoporosis, or the 'lack of backbone' energy, may be inherited, as may be the lack of love or acknowledgement. Consider that one may suffer from osteoporosis even though love from the mother was strongly present and received. However, an ancestor such as a great-grandmother may have not received the love and support, the 'backbone', she needed to feel supported.

In this situation, the perceived lack of love and lack of support energy is inherited from great-grandmother, manifesting itself in the physical realm in the future offspring, the grandchildren or the great-grandchildren. So, the work you do as the offspring to shift the associated physical deficiencies such as vitamin D deficiency or mineral deficiency must be done hand in hand with transforming negative perceptions to positive ones. Perhaps then the osteoporosis tendency will change not only in you, but also in your future generations.

As the First Nations Indigenous people believe, we have the capacity to heal seven generations back and seven generations forward. Hence, the massive generational trauma imposed on the Indigenous Peoples of Canada can potentially alter their DNA and its messages (called epigenetics) for generations to come[3]. They believe they can heal through acknowledgment, through their spiritual ceremonies and through community support[4]. Our capacity to shift our future generations' health outcomes is great.

In many of the traditional Eastern societies and religions, girls continue to be neglected, abused and not comforted by their parents, especially their fathers. It is no wonder, then, that the natural instinct of us women today in response to societal stress is to withdraw and see ourselves as small and powerless. These withdrawal responses are so deeply engraved in our family and cultural systems, as well as in our genetic imprinting, that in order to reverse these reactions, we must consciously become aware of them and admit to the reality of our history.

After honoring our ancestors and all the past has taught us, we can then consciously replace these reactions with those that are more appropriate, more positive, more capacity-building. This takes conscious effort and time as our reactions are a result of generations of cellular habit that now need to be transformed.

Various techniques such as family constellation therapy, EFT (emotional freedom technique), EMDR (eye-movement desensitization and reprocessing), and ND Square™ (a technique I have developed) can potentially be very helpful in recognizing and transforming our unwanted subconscious and negative thoughts linked to our physical symptoms to ones that are positive and situation-appropriate. Basically, the goal is to unlink the trauma memory from the physical cellular memory by consciously becoming aware of the trauma and its physical link. This helps rewire the autonomic nervous system response towards healing.

Mindful meditation is another powerful tool for optimizing and transforming the subconscious. Effective and successful mindful meditation requires a mindful choice to learn and practice such a technique. It requires a mindful intention and desire to be open to transformation, as well as an acceptance of whatever is revealed during meditation. And, finally, it takes dedication and discipline to act mindfully and practice such techniques daily. From personal experience, mindful choices, intentions and actions – leading to the regular practice of mindful meditation – undoubtedly help transform our engraved negative subconscious memories to ones with a positive impact on our physique, energy, emotions, behaviors and reactions.

Transforming the subconscious doesn't happen overnight. We must be willing to observe and acknowledge our hidden negative thoughts and behaviors and to re-pattern and re-constitute these with loving thoughts. We must replace the thought of anger with one of benevolence, the thought of hatred with one of compassion and love, and the thought of guilt with one of forgiveness and gratitude. Most importantly, to achieve such a level of transformation, we must love ourselves to the core, recognizing the beauty and the divine attributes we have been endowed with, and which we have the capacity to exhibit and inherently own.

Both personally and with my patients, I have always witnessed the wisdom in the disease process. I believe that going through the journey of chronic illness and recovery is a process of transformation. Having treated thousands of patients and partnered with these precious souls in their journey, I have witnessed them transform after their initial suffering into healthier individuals who become empowered physically, mentally and spiritually as vehicles of change for others.

If you or a loved one is suffering with a chronic illness, know that transformation and healing is possible. Our illness is an opportunity to grow in ways we never dreamt of and to become healthier in ways we never thought possible.

Reflection questions

- Think about how you can practice letting go of your ego and your desires so you can fully trust that you are on the right path – that it will lead to the right outcome. As you let go, are you aware of the stress lifting from your shoulders, your physical pain dissipating?

- Reflect on your station in life. Who are you – deep down, once you strip away all external things? What is your worth in the process of life, and what makes you unique? Do you feel isolated, unworthy or powerless? Can you link these to a trauma in your past or in your ancestry? What support do you need to unblock these stuck feelings and transform them towards oneness and nobility while letting go?

- Think about how you can practice showing yourself love and gratitude for the gifts you have been bestowed with. How can you use your purpose and your gifts to create the most authentic and fulfilled version of yourself?

Trusting my *Station*

After 30-plus years of marriage and 28 years of practicing medicine, I have learnt that I must lay all my affairs in the hands of the All-Powerful Source to reduce my stress. I am continually reminded to trust God and detach from all save Him. This does not mean I am passive in my relationships or actions. It simply means that I trust that the situation I am in will eventually guide me to the correct path.

My practice of trust and detachment means that when I am working with chronically ill patients, I use my tools to assist their healing process but, ultimately, the end result is left up to the Almighty. I give my patient all that is within me as I give up the need to have control. I stay detached from the outcomes of my desires and accept that which is the Will of God. I strive to practice this skill every day. I must constantly stay conscious of my behaviors and thoughts, let go of my ego, and then evaluate, re-evaluate and correct my thoughts and my actions accordingly.

Prayers, meditations and various emotional and energy release techniques have been a source of great aid. I remind myself that although I aim to give 100% effort to my relationships, the final outcome is not in my hands. By detaching from the end result, I am learning to be content with whatever the final outcome may be, while simultaneously being present in my relationships and my marriage.

Being submissive to His Will helps reduce my stress within my relationships. That is why our Bahá'í marriage vows were so simple, yet so powerful: "We will all, verily, abide by the Will of God."

Virtue 11

The Science of the Physical

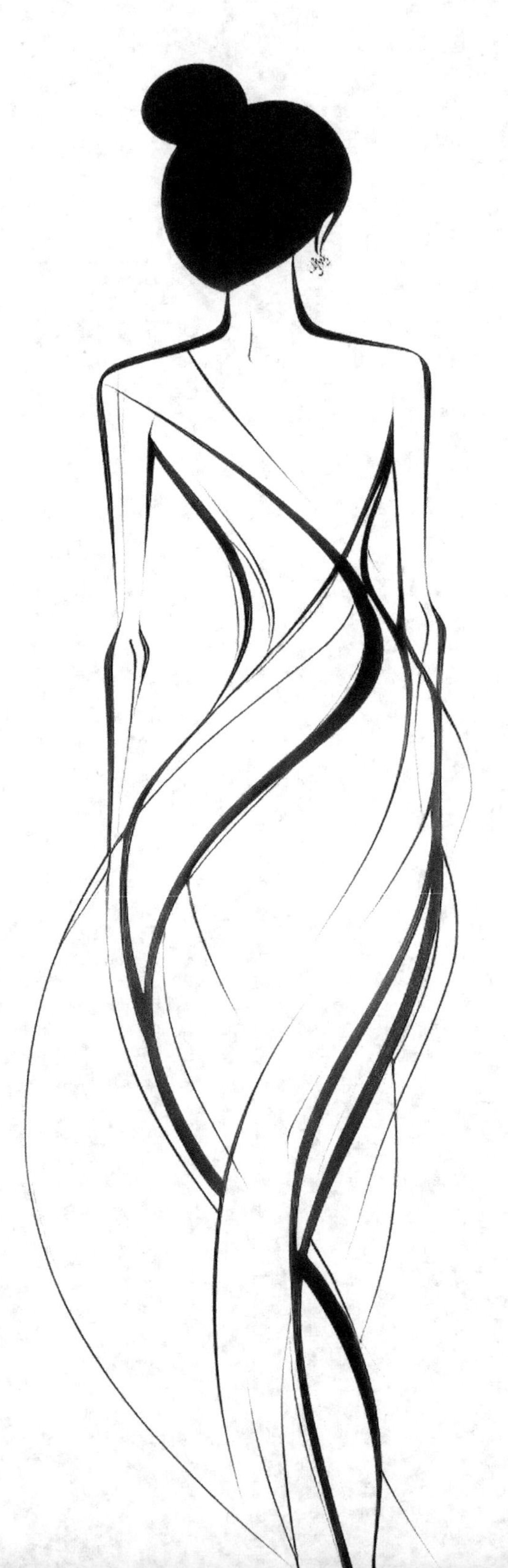

Chapter 7

Big Pharma: Friend or Foe?

"We must be like the fountain or spring that is continually emptying itself of all that it has and is continually being refilled from an invisible source."

Shoghi Effendi

I recently met an individual who had been a senior executive at a Big Pharma company for more than 35 years. During casual conversation, he told me that Big Pharma makes its profits based on the concept of "lifelong disease management".

I asked him to clarify. He said: "Big Pharma likes to make sure that diseases are not cured but only managed, so that people stay on pharmaceutical drugs for their entire lives." He continued: "For example, Metformin, a prediabetes and Type 2 diabetes drug, is for lifelong management of blood sugar." Shocked, I said to him: "So Big Pharma is not interested in finding cures for such conditions?" He replied: "We prefer to say we are in the 'disease management business'."

The executive went on to share that Big Pharma's "next big money-makers" are GLP-1 (glucagon-like peptide-1) agonist compounds like semaglutide, sold under the brand names Ozempic, Rybelsus and Wegovy – the Type 2 diabetes drugs that are now being prescribed for weight loss and endorsed by Hollywood stars as a quick fix to maintain their svelte figures. "Women who take these drugs find out very quickly that once they go off the drug, they regain the weight," he said. "So, they stay on it long-term. And that is what Big Pharma wants – for people to stay on these drugs lifelong."

The danger is that not only do patients become dependent on drugs like semaglutide, but most are often not educated on the risks associated with the use of these medications. Common side-effects of taking this type of medication include nausea, abdominal pain, malnutrition, muscle loss, hair loss and fatigue. Though the risk of heart attacks may decrease with the use of GLP-1 agonists, risks for thyroid cancer, acute pancreatitis, acute gallbladder disease, acute kidney injury and even suicidal thoughts and behavior increase.

My question: are we choosing prescription drugs because we want the quick fix? If so, we are feeding Big Pharma and making ourselves sicker as we close our eyes to the reality of the root causes of our dysfunction and the obesity/chronic disease epidemic. Or are we being ignorant, lost in the world of vanity? Is there another mindful choice we can make? I believe advanced options that address the root causes of our conditions and lead to long-term healing and graceful aging do exist, but they are not easy, and we have to pull together to achieve them. We currently find ourselves in a rat wheel spiraling down as we misdirect our future generations towards being sicker, fatter and more materialistic. Can we get ourselves off this rat wheel?

I believe we can get off the rat wheel – but it will take much conscious, collective effort. We have the capacity to naturally feel, function, and look absolutely extraordinary and beautiful, glowing with health and radiating a vibrant energy that positively affects everyone around us. Yet in the modern world, we now have access to almost anything and everything. We expect everything to be effortless, handed to us on a silver platter.

We feel entitled. We have constructed medical, social, economic, political, recreational and educational systems that have taught us to sit back and enjoy the ride. We expect education, jobs, happy relationships, money, beauty and health to fall into our laps without investing significant energy or making sacrifices. We are reluctant to work hard for our share of the rewards and have forgotten that good things don't come easily.

When we don't get what we want, we get depressed and anxious and end up on antidepressants, anti-anxiety pills – or both – as a quick fix to get what we originally sought, which is happiness. Contrary to our belief, these medications don't work either, as they come with a load of side effects and make us feel numb to the world around us. It seems we are stuck within the spikes of a wheel and keep going round and round, faster and faster. Sooner or later, we finally get thrown off the wheel even more perplexed and injured, wondering how we got here and how we are going to get fixed.

Quick Fix is a Slow Death

Being brainwashed to choose the "quick fix" is endemic in every aspect of our society. Our medical system, based on pharmaceutical greed, has brainwashed our conventional medical physicians and the public, creating a strong belief system in miracle cures that generates huge profits for the drug companies. We are conditioned to believe that the only way to cure a symptom and feel better is through prescription drugs and surgery.

Let's look at the antibiotic industry. Suffering from acne as a teenager, or even as an adult, is a common complaint. We go to the doctor who prescribes a three-month course of tetracycline, doxycycline, or spironolactone. The skin clears up and looks great, but over time a slew of other conditions may begin as a result of this relatively quick fix. Antibiotics disturb the bacterial balance in the gut resulting in an overgrowth of yeast and pathogenic bacteria, dysbiosis (an imbalance of our gut microbiome), and increased susceptibility to parasitic infections. These chronic infections lead to chronic inflammation of the gut and a dysfunctional, disrupted immune system.

Chronic inflammation leads to a plethora of issues such as fatigue, depression and anxiety, bloating and IBS, sleep problems, joint pain and body aches and – eventually – even cancer.

Your skin may look great now, but you may feel horrible. Another set of medications, such as steroids or anti-inflammatories, antidepressants or immunosuppressants, are often then prescribed for these chronic symptoms and diagnosis. These medications create a slew of new symptoms and medical problems, for which even more prescriptions are advised.

By the time you hit 50, you may be on three to six different medications and feeling sicker, more depressed and more dysfunctional than ever. You don't feel good. You look like you have significantly aged and, even worse, you are going through a divorce because of your inability to handle stress and be a positive influence in your relationship. Inflammatory bowel disease (IBD), irritable bowel syndrome (IBS), Crohn's Disease (CD), or depression may now be your new diagnosis. That's hardly a quick fix!

You may mock this example but sadly my experience has shown it to be true and more common than you may think. After decades of using antibiotics to treat acne in teenagers, research is now showing that long-term antibiotic therapy for acne significantly increases the risk of developing IBD or CD as an adult[1]. So, what is the alternative to treating acne without antibiotics? Well, instead of treating the symptoms with short-term fixes, let's investigate the cause of the acne first. The reasons for why many people get acne in the first place are listed on the next page.

Causes of Acne

- Chemical toxicity

- Chronic yeast infection in the intestinal tract

- Digestive enzyme deficiency

- Dysbiosis and parasitic infections

- Emotional and mental stress

- Food allergies and sensitivities

- Heavy metal toxicity

- Hormonal imbalances

- Hypochlorhydria or achlorhydria (low stomach acid)

- Leaky gut

- Nutritional deficiencies

Once we identify the causes for your acne and we start addressing them, you find that not only does your acne clear up, but you begin feeling emotionally and physically better. The acne was not the cause of your health problems; it was only a yellow light, a cautionary indicator, a symptom of imbalances within your being.

Some of us are beginning to realize that our belief system is based on man-made predictions, corrupt science, greed and ignorance. Something has to change so that humanity is able not only to survive but to thrive, so our civilization can continue to advance. Prescription medications and surgery are neither the initial nor the final answer. I may sound like I am anti-medications and anti-surgery. I am not.

In fact, conventional medical doctors are trained in acute care and emergency care, and they are amazing at saving lives during urgent situations. However, they rarely get any training in medical school in chronic diseases and how to manage them, the root causes of chronic disease, or non-invasive interventions such as making lifestyle changes, better nutritional choices, or herbal and homeopathic remedies.

Board-licensed naturopathic physicians receive an extra four to six years of intensive classroom and hands-on training after completing a bachelor's and pre-med degree. The first two years of naturopathic medical school are identical to that of conventional medical schooling. We study human anatomy, physiology, laboratory sciences, human biochemistry, neuroanatomy, microbiology, physical exam and pathology. The final two years, we study acute and chronic diseases, diagnosis and disease management, and the interconnectedness of the body systems – for example, how the lungs are connected to the intestines, the liver to the eyes, the gut to the brain and the adrenals to the thyroid.

We learn how to assess root causes of symptoms, and use effective evidence-based non-invasive interventions, including nutrition, botanical medicine, hydrotherapy, physical medicine, spinal and extremity manipulation, homeopathy, counseling and IV nutrition therapy. At the same time, we learn how to prescribe pharmaceutical medications and perform minor surgical interventions appropriately.

Temporary quick fixes may work for short-term solutions and instant gratification, but in the long-term they often lead to cascades of deeper, more aggressive heath issues. Using integrative and regenerative therapies to address the underlying functional imbalances to create a healthier, more vibrant, younger you – both physically, mentally and emotionally – takes time, effort, persistence and patience. But the long-term positive impact on your health and wellbeing, as well as on the health of future generations, is immeasurable.

A History of the Pharmaceutical Industry

For centuries, natural remedies such as plants, herbs, fungi, acupuncture, homeopathy, hydrotherapy, diet, lifestyle, and spiritual practices were the source of effective therapeutic healing worldwide. In Ancient Greece in 400 B.C., Hippocrates, the Father of Medicine, prescribed the active ingredient found in the bark of the white willow tree to treat fever, pain and inflammation. This ingredient is now known as salicylic acid.

The belief in natural medicine and healing continued until the early 19th century. Then in 1826, French chemist Pierre Joseph Leroux isolated the active ingredient in willow bark, called 'salicin'. And in 1897, German chemist Felix Hoffmann worked with the drug company Bayer to resynthesize and launch acetylsalicylic acid, which had been originally developed by French chemist Charles Frédéric Gerhardt in 1853[2]. By the end of the 19th century, this new drug, called Aspirin, was being sold around the world as the first anti-fever and pain-relief pharmaceutical medication[3].

Aspirin changed our world forever. It introduced us to the possibility of pharmaceutical wealth, albeit toxic wealth, and the concept of a "quick fix". I believe the powerful discovery has compromised the wellbeing of our society to this day. Ironically, rumor has it that Charles F. Gerhardt died at the age of 39, three years after discovering his chemical compound, due to poisoning from his own synthesized medication.

By 1903, the German dye company that held the patent to Aspirin set up a US subsidiary and began marketing Aspirin to physicians, hospitals and medical schools[4]. Before long, the majority of homeopathic hospitals and naturopathic medical schools throughout the US converted to pharmaceutical drug training. They had a powerful incentive: Big Pharma companies sponsored medical schools if they trained their doctors how to use their new drugs. Before long, homeopathic and naturopathic medical schools and hospitals, as well as non-invasive "natural' therapies throughout the US, were forgotten as financial enticement took precedence.

The original pharmaceutical companies were born out of the synthetic dye, textile and coal companies. The manufacturing companies provided a rich source of organic chemicals, which have become the basis of prescription and pharmaceutical medications. Phenacetin, a tablet stabilizer that is mixed with aspirin, is derived from coal tar[5] and was originally used as a stabilizer in hair-dye[6]. Despite causing severe kidney damage, Phenacetin was on the market for over 100 years before it was finally banned from the European, Australian and American markets by 1983[7].

Another example of a pain medication derived from coal tar is Acetanilide, which was synthesized in 1886[8]. The use of Acetanilide has diminished due to its unacceptable liver toxicity, but it has been replaced by its chemical offspring acetaminophen. It is most commonly known under the brand name Tylenol in the US, and as paracetamol (under the brand name Panadol) in Europe and most of the rest of the world. Acetaminophen is sold widely as the active ingredient in over-the-counter pain medication across the US, and packets of Tylenol are stocked in almost every household.

Data from the US shows that acetaminophen has now replaced viral hepatitis as the most common cause of acute liver failure and the most common cause for liver transplants in the US[9]. Incidentally, the amino acid compound NAC (N-acetylcysteine) may reverse acetaminophen-induced liver toxicity[10]. Some scientists have hypothesized a link between acetaminophen and autism[11], cognitive and behavioral disorders, and asthma in children and teens[12] because of its common use to relieve pain in infants and young children following vaccinations.

As we are all witnessing, the US population is becoming sicker and sicker, as cases of chronic disease spiral at alarmingly rates among our younger population. Nearly 50% of adults in the US population have hypertension[13], and one in ten Americans over the age of 20 have high cholesterol[14]. To "cure" this, we hand out more and more pharmaceutical prescriptions. Those most commonly prescribed in the US are statin drugs such as Atrovastin (Lipitor) to lower cholesterol, Lisinopril for elevated blood pressure, Levothyroxine for low thyroid function and Metformin for prediabetes and diabetes.

The number of individualized prescriptions for statins to treat elevated cholesterol, which is mostly treatable with diet and lifestyle, rose from 31 million users in 2008, costing $11 billion, to 92 million users in 2019, costing $22.9 billion[15]. Blood pressure, also generally a lifestyle and diet-related issue, costs the US $131 to $198 billion per year with 3.8 billion medication tablets dispensed per month in 2020[16].

You may want to pay careful attention to the contents of the next table showing some mind-blowing statistics. What mindful choices do we need to make individually and collectively to change these statistics to better our individual and societal health trajectories?

Some Scary Statistics

- Global pharmaceutical sales hit more than $1.5 trillion in 2022[17].

- The US accounted for 49% of global pharmaceutical sales in 2021, with China as the second largest global sales market at 9.4%[18].

- Around 74% of all deaths globally in 2021 were due to non-communicable (non-contagious) chronic diseases, of which the majority are preventable[19].

- Non-communicable chronic diseases and mental conditions account for 90% of the total $4.1 trillion annual healthcare costs in the US[20].

- The use of antidepressants in the US increased by 400% from 1988-1994 through to 2005-2008 and continues to exponentially increase today, with approximately 25% of women over 60 taking antidepressants[21].

- Approximately one in ten US people over the age of 12 takes antidepressants[22].

- Women take two-and-a-half times more antidepressants than men[23].

- Sales of thyroid medication in the US increased from $1.1 billion in 1997 to $3.2 billion in 2016[24].

Did you know that cholesterol and healthy fats, like omega-3 fatty acids, make up 60% of the total components of our brains and are essential to brain health? The dietary intake of omega-3 essential fatty acids, especially DHA, play a vital role in the constitution of our brain function and neurons, as well as of every cell membrane. They protect nerve cells and blood vessels, are anti-inflammatory and protect against dementia and Alzheimer's[25]. Omega-3 fatty acids improve cognition by helping the brain work less hard while maintaining brain health during aging[26].

Cholesterol is necessary for maintaining optimum function of our neurons, cellular metabolism and memories, and for healthy hormone production. Furthermore, vitamin D, bile acids, and steroid and sex hormones require healthy amounts of cholesterol to be produced. Cholesterol medications block cholesterol production, including the cholesterol produced in our brains. For instance, cholesterol medications such as Simvastatin have been shown to inhibit cholesterol biosynthesis in the brain within 12 weeks of taking the medication[27]. Meanwhile, the rate for developing Alzheimer's and dementia is the highest it has ever been in history. Alzheimer's is now the sixth-highest cause of death in the US – and more women than men are afflicted[28,29].

Is there a link between taking cholesterol-lowering medications and an increased risk of developing dementia and Alzheimer's? Do you think the high number of prescriptions for cholesterol, combined with our unhealthy lifestyle, Standard American Diet (SAD) dietary habits and our quick-fix culture, are contributing to the rate of memory loss in our population? I think more systematic, objective research is needed to verify this possibility.

Because obesity, high cholesterol, prediabetes, Type 2 diabetes and heart disease are considered lifestyle-related diseases (and not necessarily related to aging), before we blindly take medications to treat these conditions, perhaps we should first evaluate and correct our nutrition and lifestyle practices, as well as our infectious load, toxins, hormones, thoughts, stressors and our mental and spiritual states.

In 2022, the second biggest-selling prescription drug was a biological medication called Humira[30], which is approved for managing autoimmune disorders such as rheumatoid arthritis, Crohn's disease, ankylosing spondylitis, psoriasis and Hashimoto's (a thyroid autoimmune disease that is most commonly found in women). Overall, autoimmune diseases account for 8% of the US population, and 78% of those affected are women, according to the Centers for Disease Control[31]. Prescriptions for autoimmune medications such as Humira generate the biggest pharmaceutical revenues in the world — billions of dollars to be exact.

Did anyone tell you that the cause of low thyroid may be celiac disease or gluten intolerance, stress, a deficiency of B12, selenium or iodine deficiency, blood sugar dysregulation, heavy metal toxicity, hormonal imbalance, mold illness, viral infections or an autoimmune disease? I bet you no one has told you that, and especially not your conventional primary care physician.

There is something wrong here, don't you think? We are seeing that women tend to be inflicted with chronic conditions such as autoimmune disease, depression, and dementia, and women are prescribed the most expensive prescription drugs. Women also visit doctors more frequently[32] and are prescribed more medications as a result[33]: 64% of women, compared to 47% of men in the same age-bracket. In other words, Big Pharma makes trillions of dollars based on the health status of women.

To make matters worse, research cited by the Harvard Business Review[34] has shown the huge problem of giving drugs to people who don't benefit from them. It said: "Multiple studies have shown that most drugs prescribed in the US today are effective in fewer than 60% of treated patients, costing the healthcare system billions of unnecessary dollars."

It continued: "Consider the percentages of patients for whom the following widely prescribed classes of drugs are either "ineffective" or "not completely effective". At least 70% of patients who take the cardiovascular drugs known as ACE inhibitors and beta-blockers; nearly 40% of the people prescribed antidepressants; and at least 30% of both the patients given statins for high cholesterol and those given beta2-agonists for asthma. Diagnostic tests are not yet widely available to distinguish who does and who does not respond to these medications. These statistics show the great need for increased availability and utilization of such tests."

None of this adds up. We are creating more pharmaceutical drugs, investing billions of dollars in pharmaceutical research, and spending trillions of dollars on healthcare, and yet the rates of chronic disease, dementia, cancer and associated disability and deaths continue to escalate. And, don't forget, we are more depressed, forgetful and stressed than ever before. In the meantime, pharmaceutical companies are making trillions of dollars.

The great United States of America is one of the wealthiest countries in the world, but it is also one of the sickest nations in the world. There is definitely something wrong with this picture. Have we not been brainwashed to believe that pharmaceutical medications and surgery are the solutions to our health problems? Well, the numbers definitely don't seem to show it. If we continue progressing the way we have been since the discovery of aspirin, indulging in our greed for material wealth, continuing to lead high-stress lifestyles with poor dietary habits, destroying our environment because of global modernization, and creating a fear-based soulless society, our human species will become handicapped in every possible way.

To shift these statistics and to not only survive but thrive optimally, we have no other mindful choice but to transform our approach and mindset to our health and wellbeing. Not only do we need to give up our attachments to materialism and seek a balance between the science of medicine and our soul, we must also adopt plant-based whole foods nutrition and moderate active lifestyle practices, use sustainable agriculture and food production methods, attend to our earth's environment concerns and, most importantly, create a loving and unified community that feeds our being.

Since most of Big Pharma's success comes from medicating women's health, it is appropriate and necessary for women to lead such a transformation. We must start by becoming more educated about health, nutrition, and lifestyle practices conducive to bettering our total wellbeing and soul without use of prescriptions. Once we make this shift in our mindset and lifestyle, we naturally reduce our use of prescription drugs and surgery, improve our long-term health outcomes and elevate the joy and quality of our society and future generations.

When we women fully step into our role of being the Golden Gates of civilization, we have the capacity to make a powerful impact on fixing the world's health crisis. Are we ready to make that shift?

"Let warring ways be
banished from the world.
Let justice everywhere
its carpet throw.
May friendship reconcile
ancient hatreds.
May love grow from
the seed of love we sow."

Tahirih

Women Are the World's *Healers*

Women are already making a mark on the healthcare and wellness industry. We reached a turning point in 2022, when more than 56.5% of first year medical students were women for the first time in history[35]. Tipping the scale in 2022, more women doctors than male doctors graduated from medical schools[36]; in time, women will account for the biggest proportion of the world's physicians.

As long as we are true to ourselves as female healthcare providers, we are destined to shift our health and healthcare system. Women are natural nurturers, educators, caregivers and community builders; they are also empathetic, gentle, gracious, kind, compassionate, forgiving and loving. They are hungry for learning, self-education, and self-care. They are interested in disease prevention, and helping their patients establish healthier lifestyles.

It only makes sense that we women, the primary educators of future generations, must continue to educate ourselves on this path, rid ourselves of our negative self-talk, empower and support each other, and place ourselves and each other in leadership and educational positions.

We can then educate the masses, influencing and guiding other parents and their children, to make a powerful shift in the world's ailing healthcare systems. We are the Golden Gates. We have the obligation and the capacity to transform our health crisis into a health revolution for the world. In fact, it's our destiny. If we don't do this, who will?

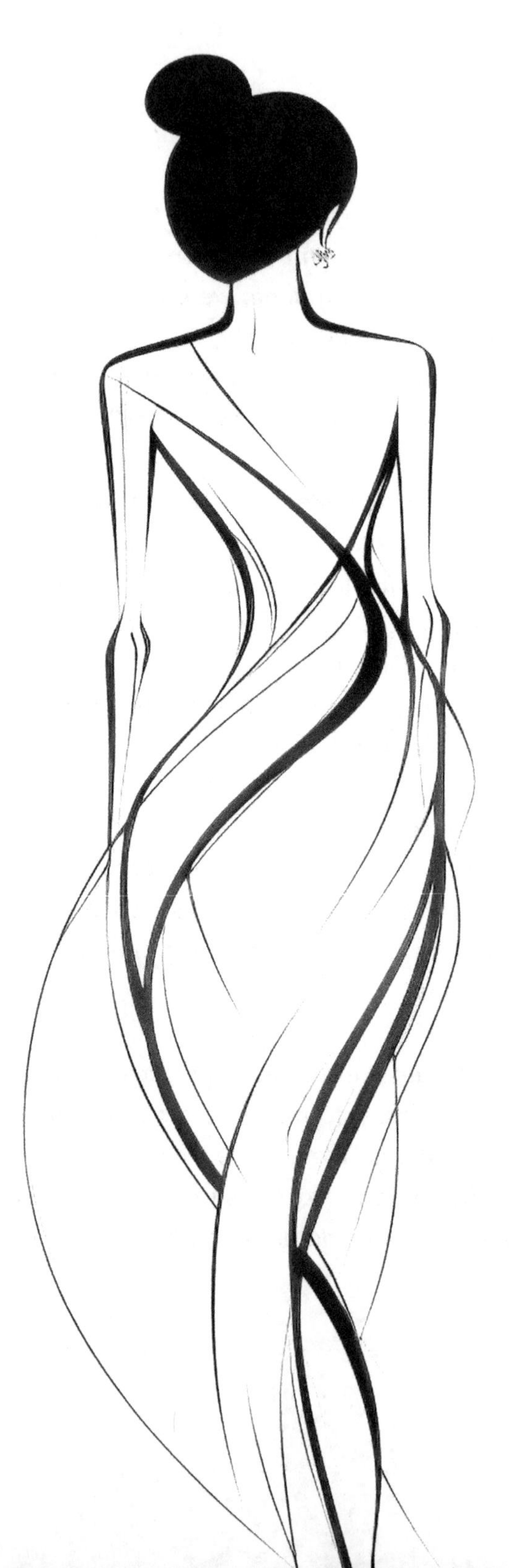

Chapter 8

Is Your Light Turned On?

"Don't you know yet?
It is your light
that lights
the worlds."

Rumi

A lamp sitting on the table is not shining. What are the possible reasons for it not working? Well, it could be because the lightbulb is out, which is easy to fix. Just replace the lightbulb. Or, it could be because the lamp is turned off, it's not plugged in, or the wiring is disconnected. Instead of changing the lightbulb straightaway, most would check first to make sure the lamp is plugged in, the wiring is connected, and the lamp switch is turned on.

This lamp illustrates the difference between western medical and functional naturopathic medical approaches to diagnosis and treatment. In western medicine, tissues and organs represent the lightbulb. If the lightbulb does not turn on, or if the particular organ malfunctions, then physicians immediately replace the lightbulb by doing surgery, or they patch it up by using prescription medications to suppress symptoms.

For example, if the gallbladder triggers excruciating pain, known as cholecystitis, conventional medical physicians are likely to recommend removing the gallbladder – even if it appears healthy on an ultrasound. However, chances are the reason the gallbladder malfunctions (the lamp is broken) is because it is not plugged in, or the switch is not turned on. In other words, the gallbladder pain may not be rooted in the gallbladder but may lie in its breakdown or inflammation caused by food, nerve pain, dysbiosis (imbalance of bacteria balance), unresolved resentment, chronic infections or other causes.

In functional naturopathic medicine, licensed physicians like myself who are well-versed in the autonomic nervous system take a different approach. We make sure all the systems of the body are plugged in to the nervous system and switched on first. This means we evaluate the body's electrical circuitry, autonomic nervous system, hormones and gut microbiome, plus the patient's emotional and nutritional status, immune system and cellular and mitochondrial function, before exchanging the lightbulb for a new one.

This may sound funny to some of you. But if you think about when a baby is born, the first check performed is to make sure the newborn's nervous system is working and all organs and systems are plugged in to the nervous system – the reflexes are working, and the baby is crying and responding to the external environment. If the baby is not, something is wrong and needs to be immediately addressed and corrected. This simple art and practice of checking reflexes and responses to stimuli – in other words, checking the autonomic nervous system function – has been generally lost in modern medicine.

The conventional model of jumping to take out an organ prior to checking the nervous system function can not only fail as a 'band-aid' treatment, but can create multiple life-threatening complications. A 2022 study showed that 31.5% of patients undergoing general surgery in the US experience post-operative complications[1], while a second study put this rate even higher – showing that 43.5% of patients suffer postoperative complications[2]. If patients had comorbidities like high blood pressure, diabetes, asthma, kidney disease or hypothyroidism, up to 82% had complications after surgery[3].

Of course, western medicine does have its merits. Life-threatening injuries and near-death calamities often require emergency medical care, prescription drugs and/or surgery. Thousands of lives are saved in the emergency room every day. But are we in a physical crisis mode every day? Do we need prescription drugs prescribed for chronic diseases as often as they are given to us? The majority of our lifespan – around 95% – is spent in non-threatening, non-critical, non-emergency mode. I believe that western medicine and functional naturopathic medicine both play a role in treating the health and welfare of humanity when used appropriately.

My guestimate is that out of every 500 or so times that the lamp button needs to be switched on, only once or twice does the lightbulb actually need changing. In other words, for every 500 symptoms and concerns we may have throughout our lifetime, we only need surgery or suppressive prescription medications a handful of times. For the vast majority of our lifetime, our symptoms and conditions can be resolved through non-invasive, holistic and naturopathic medical approaches that address the root causes and the nervous system function.

Because conventional physicians have been trained in hospitals, every symptom is either classed as life-threatening or not severe enough to warrant treatment. There is no middle ground. Symptoms that cannot be categorized into a box fall under the label: "It's all in your head." These symptoms literally are in your head, often caused by the autonomic nervous system in chaos.

The Danger Zone

Symptoms and diagnoses are like a yellow traffic-light signaling, "Caution: slow down". If we don't slow down to recognize and avoid the initial signs of danger, we may enter the "Danger Zone" later. If we suppress the symptoms, the disease processes deepen as the body continues to find an expression for its internal imbalances somewhere else.

Pharmaceutical medications often bury symptoms without correcting the underlying disease process. It is like cutting weeds at the surface of the soil without pulling out or treating the root of the weed properly. When we only treat the top layer, its buried roots and hidden seeds continue to multiply and grow quietly beneath the ground until they gain an opportunity to sprout to the surface stronger and thicker than before. Suppressing symptoms causes underlying disease processes to penetrate deeper, expand, spread and grow until they find multiple locations in the body to sprout.

This is a common scenario with cancer. When primary cancer cells are treated with chemotherapy or radiation, often the tumor may no longer be seen at the surface. But its seeds, known as cancer stem cells, continue to multiply and spread their roots, expand and grow quietly. This quiet process can sometimes continue for months or years before tumors are found once again, this time stronger, more resistant and in different organs — a process known as metastasis.

But when we treat cancer alongside its stem cells, we have a better chance of reducing its multiplication, spread and the risk of metastasis. This is one of the reasons that combining conventional cancer treatment with naturopathic oncology support often results in better outcomes than conventional therapies alone[4]. Naturopathic oncology supportive therapies aim to address cancer stem cells, their roots and their resistance to treatment.

Most of us women between the ages of 35-55 enter the danger zone as a natural phenomenon. You may already be experiencing hormonal changes: weight gain, mood swings, bloating, sleep disturbances, hot flashes, outbursts of anger, irregular menstrual cycles, hair loss, brain fog, skin changes, low libido, and fatigue, among multiple other symptoms. These symptoms may first occur before menstruation every month, but then sometimes gradually appear all month long as we approach perimenopause.

When our mood, appearance and feelings begin to change, we start thinking: "I can't believe I am turning into my mother!" When our marriages go down the drain as a result of our mood swings, personality changes and our dwindling sex life, we go to the doctor desperate for help. We leave the doctor's office diagnosed with depression and a prescription for an antidepressant and have joined the club of the 25-30% of middle-aged women depressed and on antidepressants[5]. We now have something to brag about to our girlfriends! Happy to have been given the cure and desperate to get relief from our symptoms, we start taking the prescription medications accordingly. We should start feeling better, right?

Nope! Initially, we feel less depressed, but then the side effects of the antidepressants often set in: nausea, headaches, sleep disturbances, depression, anxiety, fatigue, weight gain, and low sex drive. All the symptoms we were looking to resolve now become heightened. Our bloating and skin changes continue to get worse. Our hair keeps falling out and our heavy menstrual flow turns to hemorrhage.

We end up in the emergency room looking for more cures. This time, the doctor requests an urgent pelvic ultrasound only to find perhaps either a small growth called a polyp, a large fibroid (a benign tumor that can cause excessive bleeding or urinary problems), nothing at all, or – in rare cases – uterine cancer. The physician recommends immediate hysterectomy to surgically remove the uterus to stop the hemorrhage.

Who wants to go through surgery and all its possible complications, especially if other options exist? And when hysterectomy is performed, removing the whole uterus, the ovaries are also routinely removed. This essentially suddenly shuts down the production and presence of hormones, leaving the woman without her physical female identity as well as the hormones that are so crucial for healthy aging. If fibroids, endometriosis, polyps and cancer have been ruled out, there must be a reason for the heavy bleeding – and there must be other ways to stop it. Surgery doesn't seem to address the underlying dysfunctional root processes, only the bleeding that manifests as a symptom.

Heavy bleeding usually occurs in the perimenopausal woman as a result of an excess of estrogen and/or progesterone deficiency. We will discuss this hormone imbalance, known as estrogen dominance, in more detail in the chapters ahead. For now, know that when estrogen dominance and progesterone deficiency are corrected, heavy perimenopausal bleeding often stops.

And if a woman has a fibroid surgically removed without addressing the underlying causes, there is a high chance the fibroid will grow back. Surgery just doesn't seem right. So, what's the alternative? The fibroid acts as a reservoir for toxins and excess estrogen. Extra inflammatory hormones, such as toxic estrogen metabolites, often collect in this reservoir, as do metals, yeast, and emotions. The more estrogen-dominant the chemistry of the body, the more aggressive the fibroid. The more unresolved emotions the woman is carrying – especially around miscarriages, abortions, stillbirths and intimate relationships – the larger the toxic load and the bigger the challenge with fibroids or other pelvic conditions.

Addressing the reasons for the formation of the fibroids is key to resolving symptoms. As a naturopathic doctor, I balance and support proper hormone metabolism, treat any chronic infections and metal toxicity, apply stress management and emotional release techniques, and use proteolytic enzymes and treatments such as ultrasound therapy to address the fibroid. These methods can potentially break down or shrink the fibroids and stop the heavy bleeding, while also addressing the underlying imbalances. If this integrative approach has not shrunk the fibroids and heavy bleeding persists, then surgery may be necessary. However, if possible only the fibroid should be removed, not the entire uterus, so to reduce internal scar tissue.

Premenstrual and perimenopausal hormonal symptoms are most commonly a result of either progesterone deficiency or estrogen dominance, or both. Progesterone is often the first hormone to decline during the perimenopausal years because of its high demand during stress. And guess what: the more pregnancies one has, the more deficient the progesterone becomes and the more depression sets in. And the more stress, the more our testosterone depletes and the lower our libido becomes. Great! That is all we need after going through all those pregnancies, painful labors and sleepless nights. Does it ever end?

There is a solution to all this. A healthy menstrual cycle, without mood and physical symptoms during the perimenopausal years, requires a harmonious balance of estrogen and progesterone. When progesterone is too low, and estrogen dominates throughout most of the cycle, it feeds the uterine lining creating fibroids in some cases, or endometriosis or uterine cancer in extreme cases.

Because of the estrogen receptors in multiple areas of the body, relatively high estrogen levels increase inflammation throughout the body. Some women experience bloating, breast tenderness, moodiness, and fatigue prior to menstruation as a result of the estrogen dominance. Estrogen dominance increases the risk of conditions such as autoimmune disease, lupus, insulin resistance, obesity, diabetes, heart disease, osteoporosis, and other hormone-related cancers such as breast, lung, brain and ovarian cancers[6,7,8,9].

Taking an antidepressant doesn't change the balance between these hormones, and birth-control pills potentially make the imbalance worse. In other words, antidepressants surely do not treat autoimmune diseases, heart disease, cancer, and obesity. Oral birth control pills may suppress hormones to numb symptoms for a while, but their use may lead to other problems such as significantly increased risks of depression[10], suicide[11], blood clots[12], heart disease[13] and, perhaps, even cancer including thyroid cancer[14].

To address the underlying process of hormone imbalance and its related symptoms, the only logical solution is to improve the balance and processing of hormones: to provide the body with more progesterone and/or rid the body of its excess estrogen, and address the underlying stressors, toxicities, and nutritional deficiencies. The beauty of nature is that as hormones come into balance and as the body rids itself of toxins and inflammation, hormone-related symptoms like excessive bleeding naturally start to disappear.

Beyond balancing hormones and optimizing detoxification, we must often burrow deeper and resolve the reasons for the toxicity and the imbalances in the first place. Underneath hormone-related conditions like PMDD (premenstrual dysphoria), endometriosis, ovarian cysts and endometrial cancers, often we find not only heavy metal toxicity, but also psycho-energetic root causes. When these are addressed, the symptoms usually resolve for the long term.

This can often be a painful process of letting go of the suppressed emotions regarding past miscarriages or abortions. Sometimes, emotions or energies related to past or current intimate relationship issues are harbored in the pelvis and need to be released. It is not an easy process, but a necessary one if we are to close the chapter of the cycling years as menopause approaches to lead us into new territories of discovery and opportunities for personal growth.

As all this heals, the yellow cautionary light, the one that was signaling pain or imbalance, is no longer needed. Mood, skin, hair, brain function, sleep cycles and hormonal cycles begin to heal and normalize – not to mention libido and relationships. Most importantly, the risks for cancer and future chronic diseases drop as the chronic inflammatory processes settle without suppression. Keep in mind that your particular situation may not be as simple as the above scenario. It is best to consult a licensed naturopathic functional medical doctor for a comprehensive evaluation and personalized treatment of your particular condition.

Another common condition that often progresses into the danger zone because of lack of root cause assessment and treatment is when the metabolic system develops Type 2 diabetes. Diabetes does not occur overnight. Before diabetes sets in, we typically see decades of poor health and lifestyle choices and associated health issues. These include mismanaging stress, frequent yo-yo dieting and meal-skipping, high intake of carbohydrates and processed food, lack of sleep, overworking leading to burnout, long-term alcohol intake, continual exposure to food allergies and intolerances, undiagnosed chronic yeast, parasitic or viral infections, and problems assimilating and digesting food and absorbing its nutrients.

Women (and men) fighting these lifestyle conditions often experience enlarged abdominal girth, cholesterol issues, weight gain, fatigue, sexual dysfunction and blood-pressure changes — collectively known as metabolic syndrome, or prediabetes. In many, fatty liver may be the only sign of insulin resistance or prediabetes. If only we would recognize these indicators as the first stages of progression to diabetes and address their underlying lifestyle, environmental, and emotional causes before they become a big deal, we would prevent the formation of the one of fastest-growing chronic conditions in the world among adults and children.

Although the majority of cases of diabetes are Type 2 diabetes, 60% of new cases of Type 1 diabetes occur before the age of 30[15]. According to the Centers for Disease Control and Prevention, 11.6% of the US population (38.4 million people) have diabetes and 48.8% of adults over 65 have prediabetes. In 2022, diabetes cost the United States $413 billion in direct medical costs and lost productivity[16].

Beyond the Conventional Mindset

Functional or integrative naturopathic physicians view symptoms as a manifestation of the internal imbalances that are present before life-threatening events occur. I define integrative naturopathic medicine as: "An integration of evidence-based medical systems from around the world that, when combined, form a powerful healing system that treats the whole person — body, mind, emotions, and soul — in the quest for optimal health and wellness."

According to the naturopathic medicine philosophy, the body, mind, spirit and emotions have the innate capacity to heal when obstacles to cure are removed and the system is instead provided with all that it needs (e.g. nutrition, oxygen, love, etc.). The result opens the pathway to gaining coherence in life.

Board-licensed naturopathic medical physicians believe that the whole person is made up of interdependent parts, and that if one part is not working properly then all the other parts may be affected. In this way, negative imbalances (physical, mental, emotional, or spiritual) can negatively affect the overall health, while positive forces can promote physical, mental, emotional and spiritual health and regenerative processes.

According to the six principles of naturopathic medicine, the body is endowed with the wisdom to heal itself with minimal interventions, by using tools provided primarily in nature and with the predominant intention of causing no harm. The root causes of disease and suffering must be identified and corrected using patient education as a powerful tool to prevent disease. The practice of disease prevention and education is the foundation for the most desirable method of restoring the body to total health, reconnecting with the environment, food, lifestyle, mind and spirit, and optimizing youthful aging.

If we continue to mismanage chronic diseases, like prediabetes, and avoid treating the underlying root causes, then not only will individuals and families suffer greatly as they age, we also jeopardize the wellbeing of our future generations.

Ladies, my friends, it is time to acknowledge and treat the root causes of chronic diseases so prevalent in our society. Let's recognize the role that our materialistic desires and quick-fix approaches have played in the evolution of our sick society, and let's start to shift it by healing ourselves and elevating ourselves to higher levels by turning our light on. Is your light on?

<u>Case study: Addressing the Root Cause</u>

A 63-year-old patient, called Josie, came to our clinic complaining of severe recurrent gallbladder pain. On evaluation, conventional doctors did not find a diseased gallbladder but decided to surgically remove it anyway to relieve Josie's pain.

During the procedure, Josie's bile duct was accidentally severed and a second emergency procedure was performed to correct the life-threatening surgical error. Within a few months, Josie needed a liver transplant to fix the complications caused by the second surgery. Further rounds of surgery followed to correct multiple complications – but the initial gallbladder pain had still not gone away. In fact, the pain was so bad that Josie had to be rushed to the emergency room every couple of months.

Ten years after the initial surgery to remove her gallbladder, Josie was still in pain and she had started to suffer from severe itching all over her body. Her skin had become so sensitive that even the light touch of clothing was unbearable. Even though Josie was taking multiple medications to stop the pain and itching, the pain became more frequent and she developed new symptoms – jaundice and severe fatigue. Unable to work and confined to her home, eventually depression set in for Josie too.

At this point, Josie came to our clinic. Our comprehensive naturopathic evaluation revealed multiple chronic infections in the bile and pancreatic ducts, scar tissue from surgeries and emotional stressors. We also diagnosed Josie with digestive malabsorption, leaky gut, mitochondrial dysfunction, mast cell activation syndrome, hormonal imbalances, detoxification and methylation issues, and autonomic nervous system dysfunction.

To finally relieve her pain, we started a holistic treatment plan. We gave Josie intravenous doses of palladium and alpha lipoic acid complex, alongside intravenous artesunate (the active ingredient of the artemisinin herb used for malaria, severe infections and cancer). Josie's treatment plan also involved dietary modifications, emotional clearing, nutritional supplements, digestive enzymes, detoxification therapies, peptide and ozone therapies, IV nutrient therapy and neural therapy for her physical and emotional scars.

Within a few months, the frequency and severity of Josie's abdominal pain significantly decreased and finally resolved. Her generalized body pain and itching gradually went away too, her jaundice disappeared and her energy improved. She finally began healing physically, emotionally and mentally. She returned to work.

In this case, addressing the multiple root causes of Josie's symptoms resolved her pain, itching, jaundice and fatigue while reducing the emotional burden she was carrying. When Josie returned to her daily activities, she became an inspiration for her family and friends.

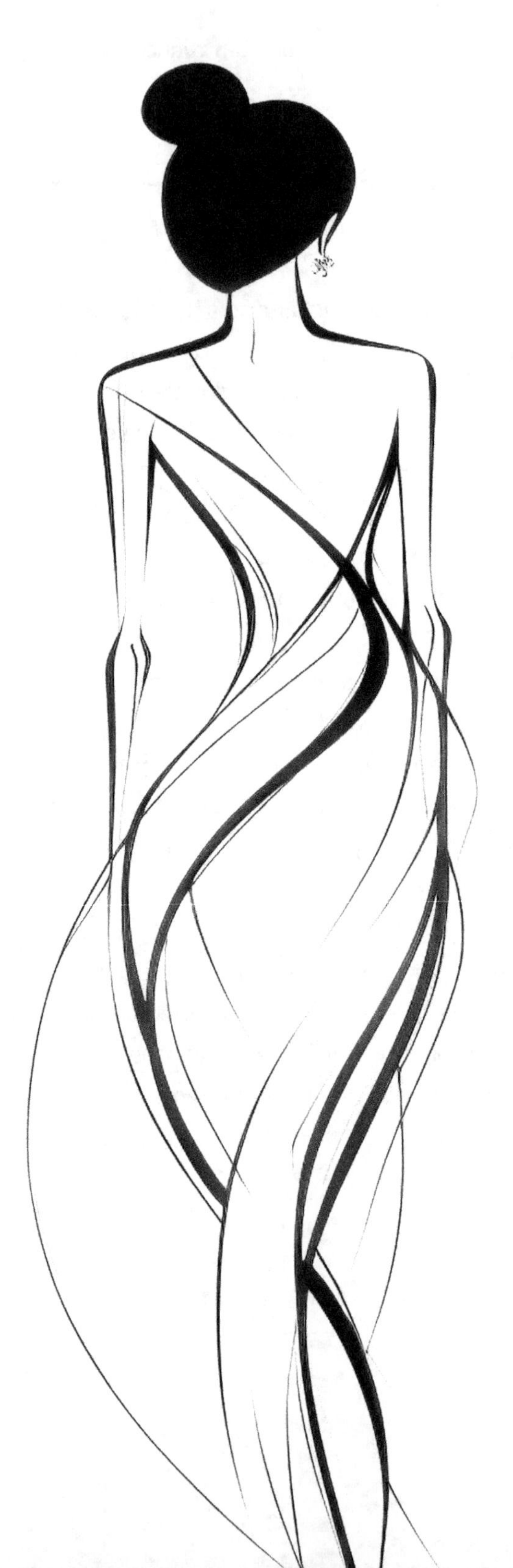

Chapter 9

The Power of Being Plugged In

"In the beginning of his
human life, man was
embryonic in the world of
the matrix. There he received
capacity and endowment
for the reality of human
existence. The forces and
powers necessary for this
world were bestowed upon
him in that limited condition."

'Abdu'l-Bahá

Our nervous system is our main power supply. Its electrical signals innervate every organ, muscle, blood vessel, tissue, and system in our bodies. It interacts with the world within and the world beyond us. It impacts and is impacted by our emotions, our microbiome, our thoughts, our senses, our beliefs, our emotional heart and our spirit.

Without a functioning nervous system, we cannot walk or talk, our heart won't beat, our skin can't sweat, and we cannot think and apply our thoughts into actions. The nervous system provides vital information so our bodies can interact with others and our environment. It also receives information from our cells and organs and feeds this back to our mind. In short, we need a healthy and balanced nervous system to be physically, mentally and emotionally sound.

A nervous system that does not function properly can throw our thoughts and emotions into disarray. It can make our immune system more susceptible to viral infections or behave chaotically, as we see in patients with mast cell conditions, like chronic hives and migraines, or autoimmune diseases. A dysfunctional nervous system can also lead to digestive problems, inflammation, blood sugar and hormonal imbalances, sleep disturbances, or keep us in a state of chronic disease or cancer. Other examples of physical manifestations of a disrupted nervous system include tingling, numbness, headaches, dizziness, fatigue, heart palpitations, sweating or bloating. In extreme circumstances, we may suffer from seizures and mental illness.

When our autonomic nervous system is functioning well, our cells heal, our mental clarity improves, our immune system becomes stronger, and our digestive tract restores to better assimilate and absorb food and nutrients. Our emotions begin to regulate. In short, chronic disease begins to abate. Though our emotions affect our nervous system and our nervous system reaction influences our emotions, we have the capacity to consciously regulate our nervous system and emotions to ameliorate our physical symptoms.

From my own experience, I have learnt that I can shift my abdominal bloating by meditating and focusing on letting go of the stressors I may be containing within my sympathetic nervous system in my belly. First, I visualize and focus on the tension in my belly. Then, I name the emotion(s), like worry, insecurity, rejection and so on that I associate with that tension as I feel into it while placing my hand on my abdomen. I may see a memory, a color or an associated image with that emotion. I consciously accept that emotion and that memory. I then ask my nervous system/belly what virtue(s), what light do I seek to assist to replace that negative emotion or darkness. The body responds as long as I am patient and open to answers.

The answer for me may be: I am worthy and noble, I am love, I am grace, I am joy, and/or I am at one. Such positive thoughts, emotions and affirmations activate the parasympathetic nervous system and replace the sympathetic stress response. I then acknowledge and consciously thank and honor the stressor, the image or negative emotion, and say 'goodbye' to it as I throw it into the universe with my hands and begin to replace it with a new positive emotion as I tap on acupuncture points. I literally watch my bloating begin to vanish. Then I write down that affirmation and consciously speak it, think it and tap it into my nervous system over and over again for several days and weeks until my system rewires to a new way of thought process, to a new calming way of being. This takes repetition and practice. As Aristotle said: "We are what we repeatedly do. Excellence, then, is not an act, but a habit."

It is quite incredible to witness how our body can present itself in different ways physically in response to the nervous system's stress reactions. An extensive network of communication exists between our emotions and the nervous, immune, hormone and lymphatic systems. Amazingly, we can control our blood pressure, heart rate, immune response, some physical symptoms and stress response through our conscious awareness and thoughts. The evidence comes from the field of psychoneuroimmunoendocrinology, initially identified in 1936[1], which shows that the interactions between these systems are highly influenced by psychological factors and linked to immune system-mediated diseases.

For instance, when we are chronically sleep-deprived due to perceived emotional stress, our stress hormones, sympathetic nervous system and immune system activate increasing inflammation, and leading to higher risk of chronic disease and cancer. Inversely, we have the ability to transform our cellular, immune, psyche, hormonal and nervous system responses (and thereby disease processes) by meditation, stress-relieving therapies like acupuncture and biofeedback therapy, and our conscious awareness and positive virtuous thoughts[2].

The Matrix

Throughout the last couple of decades, a surge in the growth of medical and scientific research focusing on the mind-body connection and quantum healing has brought a new perspective to identifying possible causes of disease and new solutions to cure them.

Cell biologist and author Bruce Lipton PhD explains the importance of quantum energy and healing in depth in his book *The Biology of Belief*. His thesis is that the electromagnetic field we unknowingly generate by our thoughts, beliefs, emotions and behaviors sends out unconscious vibrations that affect the way our cells heal and how others respond to us. I agree with his hypothesis and have witnessed its miracles thousands of times with patients and myself.

Our field may be either positively or negatively charged. It releases an electromagnetic wave rippling throughout space, or what has now been identified as the matrix. Most of us don't know much about the matrix, yet we are immersed in it. It is within us. It is around us. And we cannot function without it. It sounds like something out of this world and, well, it is. The matrix is space. It is the space between two people. It is the space between two cells. It is the space where a complex network of communication signals and exchanges occur, where toxins collect, and where the regulation of the immune, psychological, endocrine and nervous systems takes place[3].

The matrix is where emotions speak and the cells listen. It is the space where tissue damage and repair take place, and the space through which metabolic wastes are eliminated and the cells are nourished. The matrix intermeshes within itself and the world around us. Life began and continues in the matrix. It is the environment, the milieu, the terrain where cells live and where we live. The matrix is even, perhaps, where the mind is found.

According to Daniel Siegel MD, clinical professor of psychiatry at UCLA School of Medicine, the mind is not contained within the brain, as neuroscientists may argue. The mind is greater. He defines the mind as being "an embodied and relational process that regulates the flow of energy and information"[4]. Without the matrix, there would be no life and, certainly, there would be no joy, excitement, love, or passion. Without the matrix, we would be void of a mind.

The matrix is like the complex intermesh of the global internet. It is an intricate body-wide transmission system of networks that is not necessarily visualized but is deeply sensed. It is like the electromagnetic field created by the planets, propelling them to move rhythmically through space on their own orbit paths in the solar system. Just like the planets, our cells communicate with each other through the matrix. Signaling chemicals associated with the nervous system function, called neuropeptides, are released from one cell and picked up by another, creating order within the matrix and our body.

The matrix is an open energy system, interlinked with the network of the world outside. It senses the information from inside our being and relays it to others and the world and vice versa. The matrix is where the exchange of both metabolic and energetic signals happens. It is cyberspace for the immune system, the nervous system, the endocrine (hormone) system, the psycho-emotional system, the microbiome and the soul. It is where these six systems meet to communicate and exchange information.

It is here in the extracellular matrix (the matrix outside each cell) where either health or disease begins. Research by Ricker's quoted in Alfred Pischinger's book, *Extracellular Matrix and Ground Regulation for a Holistic Biological Medicine*, confirmed the theory of healing through the synchronicity of energetic, biochemical and physiological exchange in the matrix that Hippocrates, Galen, Paracelsus, Avicenna and Hahnemann had hypothesized centuries ago. Environmental toxins such as chemicals, metals, pesticides, herbicides and prescription medications deposit in the matrix, producing an electrical charge that negatively affects our physiology, cellular energy, hormones and nervous system.

The biochemical interaction of chemicals produced by the neuro-endocrine system (the nervous and hormone systems) then create either positive or negative ionic charges. Our thoughts and our subconscious, both positive and negative, also produce a charge within the matrix. As all these different components are stored and released in the matrix interface, a net positive or negative charge is generated, creating either health or disease within our cells.

The Law of Resonance

The frequency of the wave of substances becomes important in bio-energetic medicine, including homeopathy, acupuncture and European Biological Medicine. When two substances with the same charge and frequency of wavelength come together, they resonate. In homeopathy, we call this the Law of Similars. In European bio-energy medicine, we label it the Law of Resonance. When we use this technique for healing, we use effective medicines, foods, nutrients, herbs, remedies and other therapies that resonate with the patient's nervous system, emotional system, psycho-neuroendocrine system, immune system, and the communication network within the matrix. This resonance intensifies and confirms the healing process.

However, medications, herbs, nutrients, foods and therapies which do not resonate can potentially create negative effects. In Western medicine, we call this a 'side effect'. The non-resonating therapies may cause harm or delay the healing process of cells and the matrix due to the accumulation of opposite charges and chemicals.

Communication between people is not only through our five senses (visual, olfactory, verbal, somatosensory (touch) and auditory), but is beyond the tangible too. We often refer to this intangible sense as 'the sixth sense', which consists of the Law of Resonance, the knowing of our electromagnetic field. Our thoughts produce an electromagnetic field and shift the electric charge in the matrix. Our imagination, memories and beliefs can do the same.

If these thoughts are positive, they can induce electromagnetic changes that have a positive impact on our matrix and our nervous system to promote good health. Positive thoughts, such as believing that you are an effective and powerful speaker as you go up on stage, create strength, vitality and courage. They will give you a stronger voice and you'll radiate energy that captivates the audience. Positive, self-affirming thoughts change the electromagnetic field of our nervous system and our matrix towards strengthening our body and its performance.

But negative emotions and thoughts, including negative self-talk, generate electromagnetic charges that weaken our physical function. They directly release neurochemicals within our matrix that trigger a fight or flight response in our body, placing it under stress. For instance, when you think of a past trauma, or fear of failure, as you get up on stage to present, you may feel physical symptoms of butterflies, shaking limbs and heart palpitations. Your voice may tremble.

Our capacity to influence these electromagnetic changes within our system and cells is so powerful that they affect the expression of our genetics and DNA[5]. This is known as the science of epigenetics. In other words, we have the capacity to turn genes on or off through our electromagnetic state (and our thoughts)[6] and its impact on the matrix, the nervous system, neuro-endocrine chemicals and more.

Furthermore, distance does not matter when these electromagnetic fields interact, because we can be aware of people's situations, traumas, joys, successes and conflicts on a subconscious level. You may feel the sadness of your friend's loss in another country, or you may feel the stress in your neighbors' marriage even though they haven't shared this with you. You may even feel the presence of your grandmother's soul after she has passed on. This is called compassionate empathy[7], a feminine quality that helps us be compassionate and relate to others.

Have you ever noticed how, when you enter a room of people, you have an instinctive sense of whom you do and don't want to talk to? Your field almost has a mind of its own. It knows where to go to be happy and to stay away from those who will make you sad or upset. (By the way, those people who push your buttons the wrong way often represent a signal for you to look within to heal that which needs healing). The total net charge of others produced by their toxins, emotional state, nervous system and microbiome etc. will either resonate or repel with yours, helping you unconsciously decide where you would rather be and who you would rather talk to.

I experience the Law of Resonance multiple times throughout the day with my husband, daughters, close friends, my team, and my patients. Even though we may be physically apart or on two different continents, we can still experience the Law of Resonance. After comparing notes, we often realize how in sync we are with the others' thoughts. When I am present with patients, I intentionally become aware of the electromagnetic field produced by their matrix in order to feel what they are feeling and to understand what needs to alter to allow them to heal.

I use this Law of Resonance in conjunction with my medical knowledge as a guide to direct me towards what laboratory tests we may need to run, what root causes we may need to investigate, or which therapies we may need to incorporate. I then back up my 'bio-energetic' findings with laboratory tests.

In the meantime, the patient often senses and comes into synchronicity with the healthier, healing and positive matrix of the physician and the healing energy of the clinical space. The exchange of atoms and electromagnetic fields that takes place within milliseconds of coming into the other's field has profound effects on healing.

Through my own observations as a physician, I have witnessed the immediate shift that occurs in a patient's facial color, mood, pupillary reflex, strength of voice and sense of wellbeing when I enter the patient's room in a happy, compassionate, empathetic and positive state. I have seen near-death patients wake up when a positive friend or relative walks in and brings them joy and hope. The healing that occurs within those few seconds of positive interaction is often more powerful than any pill or surgery. And thus, their healing journey begins.

Regulate the Electricity!

We have two types of nervous systems: the central nervous system which includes the brain and the spinal cord, and our peripheral nervous system. Our peripheral nervous system includes the voluntary (somatic) nervous system (SNS) and the involuntary (autonomic) nervous system (ANS). Our SNS involves the voluntary control of our muscles, for example, while the ANS includes the sympathetic and parasympathetic nervous systems. The ANS plays a key role in regulating our cells, our blood pressure, our immune function, our digestion, our hormones and our health.

The nervous system, our electrical wiring, must send out signals systematically and rhythmically in order for our cells and matrix to stay healthy. Toxins, malnutrition, stress, dehydration, injuries, scars, spinal misalignments, and emotional and spiritual obstacles all interfere with our nervous system's regulation. They cause our nervous system to malfunction, thus interfering with the body's innate healing process so we head towards disease. If we identify and remove interferences to healing, the nervous system's signals become activated and regulated. When we provide the body with its necessary building blocks, release scars, realign the spine, muscles and joints while eliminating all that it sees as negative toxins, and center ourselves with our spiritual core and breath, our physical, biochemical, mental and emotional levels often return to healthy balanced levels. The disease process appears to reverse and our symptoms dissipate as a result.

Disease results from long-term accumulation of underlying dissonance within the biochemical, physiological and emotional processes. For instance, cancer does not appear overnight. Before we see signs of cancer, there have been years of toxicity, detoxification malfunction, malnutrition, cellular and mitochondrial damage, immune and autonomic nervous system malfunction, hormonal disruptions, chronic infections, disorder within the matrix or emotional stress – or a combination of these factors.

Once a cancer cell is born, it takes a minimum of three to five years of cell replication before radiologists can see the pool of cancer cells as a 1cm "mass" on ultrasounds, X-rays, mammograms, or MRI and CT scans.

If cancer cells are not visualized on imaging or detected in blood, cancer is often ruled out or announced to be "in remission", despite the presence of undetectable, yet circulating, cancer cells and its associated cancer stem cells. Conventional medical diagnosis often bases its findings on visual science. If a disease cannot be seen in blood, urine, stool or on imaging, it does not exist. Sadly though, by the time disease has been detected by conventional western medical standards, the cancer has progressed too far and may be untreatable.

Our body, thoughts and nervous system then activate the survival 'fight-and-flight' response as our conventional medical team reacts to the disease with similar aggression and urgency, justifying treatment by invasive and extreme conventional methods such as surgery and chemotherapy.

It is like firemen coming to a fire that is now raging. Their only recourse is to pour massive amounts of water over the fire to calm it down. But if we had reached the fire when it was just starting or, better yet, prevented it from starting in the first place, we would not be in an emergency situation dealing with a massive fire that needs an aggressive solution.

In my integrative or functional naturopathic medical practice, we attempt to get to the fire before it starts, or early on before it turns wild. We use changes in the electrical or electromagnetic system (especially those within the matrix) along with functional and physiological imaging and laboratory tests (like the Galleri Early Detection Cancer test[8]), to establish the basis for subtle physiological, biochemical and cellular changes in the cells that may signal the start of a fire, or an environment that may be conducive to the start of a fire. In modern medicine, distortions in the electrical system may be identified and measured via ECG (electrocardiogram) for the heart, EEG (electroencephalogram) for the brain, and EEG (electromyography) for the muscles.

We use electrodermal testing (EDA), a new device that measures the electrical system of the skin. EDA testing is based on the premise that changes in emotions are linked to specific patterns of the autonomic nervous system activity. This means we can monitor patients' emotional health by analyzing psycho-neuro-immunological data collected through measuring the activity of their autonomic nervous system.

Thanks to recent breakthroughs, EDA devices are now the most promising method of measuring a patient's stress response, emotions and the sympathetic activity of the nervous system[9]. This is key to treating disease, because our electrical system – especially our autonomic nervous system – is our primary system for regulating activities and reactions within our bodies. Tracking changes in blood pressure, heart rate, bowel movements, body temperature, sweating and emotions is the first step in identifying and measuring a patient's health status.

During perimenopause, for instance, the disruption of the autonomic nervous system due to the decline in hormones results in distressing physical symptoms such as hot flushes, mood swings, skin rashes, heart palpitations, sleep disorders and digestive troubles. The autonomic nervous system dysregulation further leads to anxiety, mood swings and depression and, in turn, such emotions cause changes to the hormone and the autonomic nervous systems. It is a vicious cycle that can be measured using EDA devices. Once we work on regulating the autonomic nervous system function through various techniques that transform the physiology, emotions and thought processes, the woman's perimenopausal symptoms often resolve.

However, when the nervous system is confronted by declining hormones and is not trained to re-regulate itself physiologically and emotionally, ultimately changes in the microbiome (the colony of bacteria in the gut) set in, fueling further imbalance. Over time, changes in the microbiome may lead to other conditions such as acid reflux, constipation, abdominal pain, IBS (irritable bowel syndrome) and inflammation during pre-menstruation or perimenopause. If left unaddressed, these symptoms initiate a whole new slew of chronic conditions.

In my integrative naturopathic practice, evaluating the ANS (which I also referred to as our bio-energetic system), plus a woman's emotional and spiritual state, takes precedence over, but does not replace, conventional laboratory and imaging analysis. We use techniques and functional medicine tests to assess the function of the autonomic nervous system, hormones, neurotransmitters, neuropeptides, cells, tissues and organs, emotions and the subconscious and their interactions with each other. This gives us the information to discover any imbalances and dysfunctions in the body before these imbalances lead to a more serious disease diagnosis.

In this way, naturopathic medicine provides genuine preventative medicine. For example, physiological heat patterns visualized on thermography can show early signs of angiogenesis (blood vessel feed to cancer cells) often before a mass can be detected by conventional imaging systems. When we incorporate preventative naturopathic medical techniques as part of our first steps to health, we can potentially reverse the symptoms and progression of disease naturally and optimize function while slowing aging.

We evaluate, correct and regulate early-stage signals the body is sending to alarm us of primal dysfunction. We evaluate and correct the disturbed milieu, the body's troubled terrain, signaling disease growth. We evaluate and personalize treatment to address the woman's autonomic nervous system, hormonal imbalances, toxic loads, genetic mutations, emotional stressors, nutritional deficiencies, cellular and mitochondrial dysfunction, chronic inflammation and stealth infections to consciously create a graceful aging process that will lead to ultimate joy and wellbeing.

A New Blueprint

Let's look at where we need to begin to help ourselves re-establish our health and to promote graceful aging. The bulk of our chronic and recurrent symptoms, syndromes, discomforts, suffering and diseases stem from our learnt lifestyle practices and, more specifically, a toxic mindset and negative emotional baggage that trigger damaging mutations in our cells and changes in their function.

The sickness of our bioenergetic, neuro-endocrine, emotional and spiritual states affects our matrix, our ANS, our cellular milieu, and all our bodily systems, making us chronically ill. We have the power to prevent chronic disease and promote healing within our cells during our lifetime. However, we need a personalized and systematic therapeutic plan that addresses the totality of our mind, body, soul and spirit.

On a daily basis, consider consciously practicing clearing any emotional baggage and epigenetic stressors that burden your nervous system and matrix and, most importantly, block your access to growth opportunities for your soul. By correcting our individual physiological imbalances and nourishing our system, our being ultimately begins to heal itself. In short, we need to create a new personalized blueprint that will guide us towards health and wellbeing.

This new masterplan involves initiating and practicing new habits founded on a constructive and auspicious mindset. As we opt for mindful choices, positive and loving intentions, healing virtues, and daily lifestyle practices designed to transform our relationship with food and nutrition, our inner self, our essential relationships, and our environment, we become aware of and elevate our fundamental desires, our vibrational frequencies, and our emotional and subconscious thoughts. Ultimately this will help to regulate our autonomic nervous system to give healing messages to our cells.

Daily prayer, meditation, and reflection must go hand in hand with consciously adopting a posture of learning and service. These will become our spiritual tools to feel happy and joyful, allowing us to begin our healing journey. We must learn to love ourselves, to be compassionate and patient with our journeys, to replace our fears with love and to share our love with others. We will then see how others' happiness is ours too, and how our joy positively affects them. We will learn that maximizing the power of our feminine gifts, such as our empathy, nurturing, gentleness, compassion and patient qualities, is the key to our wellbeing, and to the wellbeing of our community and our global society.

We will also notice that the roots of chronic disease are the blocks and impediments we have subconsciously or consciously created for ourselves — all these blocks stress our nervous system, our matrix and our cells. We will become aware that the solutions are so simple, and yet we make it so very difficult for ourselves to heal, to transform and to revolutionize the health of our body, mind, spirit, and soul.

The powerful forces within our matrix show how our feelings, thoughts and behavior significantly affect our individual and universal wellbeing. For the sake of our own health, and the health of those around us, it is vital that we each seek to make mindful choices, think positively and practice loving thoughts and moral uprightness in all aspects of our lives. Healing begins with each of us individually.

This is one more step towards recognizing that we are Golden Gates. Not only do women have the power to create a health revolution, we have the power to transform our DNA to unleash our cells towards more youthful aging and pave the way for healthier future generations.

Case Study: Biofeedback Therapy

When we become conscious of the control of our autonomic nervous system (ANS), we can influence how our cells function.

Biofeedback therapy works at this level. When we use biofeedback techniques, we become aware of and control our breathing, heart rate and blood pressure. We also become aware of how the autonomic nervous system responds to physical changes, and how this influences the health of our immune, heart, lung and digestive systems.

A 24-year-old woman who came to my clinic had a lot of anger, anxiety, sleep disturbances, weight issues, constipation, and hormonal imbalances. It was evident right from her first visit that the core issue was her stressed nervous system due to residual anger from being bullied as a teenager. She was holding on to extra weight and constantly feeling anxious and unsafe because of the shock of the trauma she had experienced.

At the clinic, we helped her reach awareness about the connection between her mental state and her physical symptoms, which was the foundation of starting her healing journey. This awareness helped her to process and let go of the past trauma she was holding on to in her abdomen, and to consciously calm the nervous system's fight-and-flight response by replacing her thoughts and emotions with more positive ones.

As a result, her weight, insomnia and hormonal issues improved as she regained the health of her nervous system. She soon was able to wean off her anti-anxiety medication and lose excess abdominal weight. Her digestion and sleep also improved significantly. She now is back to working and contributing to the welfare of her family and community.

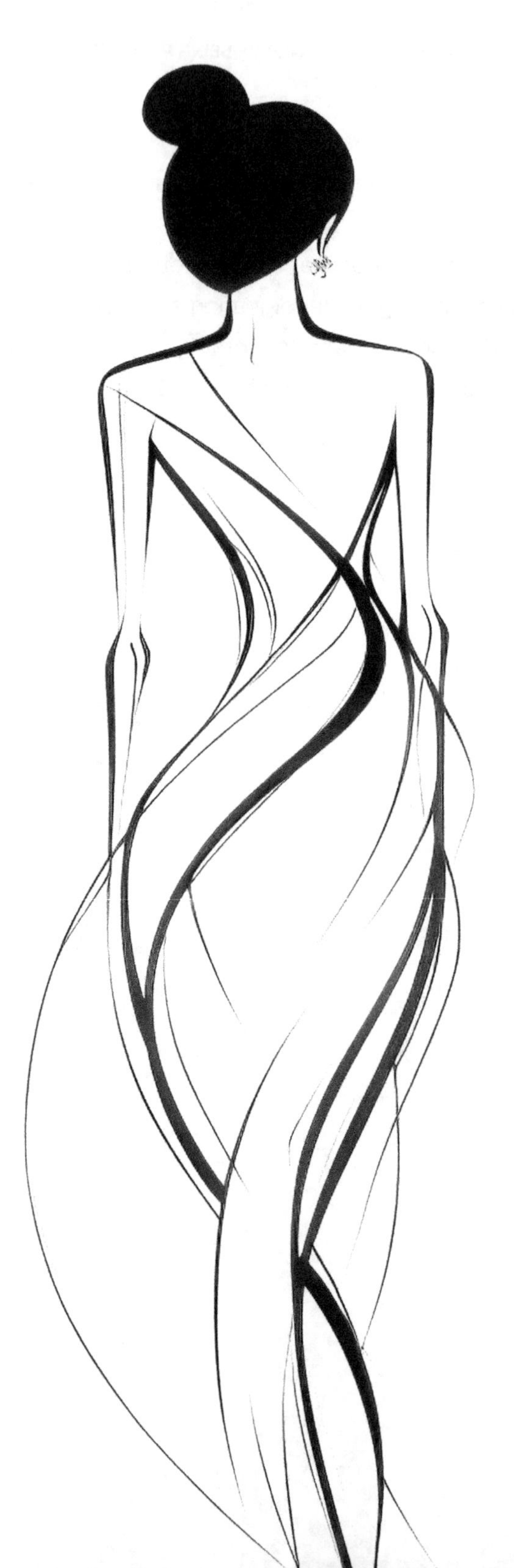

Chapter 10

Release to Rejuvenate

"The more healthful
his body, the greater will
be the power of the spirit
of man; the power of the
intellect, the power of
the memory, the power
of reflection would
then be greater."

'Abdu'l–Bahá

How are you feeling by now? Are you feeling elated and inspired or are you feeling tired, depressed, heavy and bloated? Are your PMS or perimenopausal symptoms feeling out of control? Are you suffering from low libido, brain-fog and anxiety? How about hot flashes, erratic moods and just feeling blah? Oh, and those tiresome joints… so stiff and painful whenever you try to get up. Going for a walk becomes a real chore – and all that may be churning in your head is, "All I need is sugar or chocolate." Or perhaps it's: "Where is that wine bottle? I need a drink." So, what is it that is making you feel so sluggish, so heavy and so downright yucky?

The answer is simple: toxins! Toxins are all around us, passed on to us, created by us and found within us. Yes, you heard me correctly: we intentionally and unintentionally create toxins within our cells. Most of the time, we are not even aware of the toxins we produce or are exposed to. Every time our mind perceives stress, stress hormones like cortisol released to combat our stress, lead to toxic chemical build-up in our cells and in our organs. We cannot get away from our toxic world completely. The food we consume, the medications and drugs we ingest, the pesticides we absorb from the environment, the exhaust we breathe while sitting in the car.... all these toxins filter into our bodies and must filter out.

How about the cellphone we use, and the make-up we apply? All contain toxins that are absorbed into our cells, activating more biochemical detoxification processes in our cells and organs to fight the toxic exposure. Did you know that more than 60% of our clothing is synthetic textiles made from petrochemical products?[1] Your socks are made from plastic and could be loaded with Bisphenol A (BPA), an endocrine-disrupting chemical (EDC) that can be absorbed through your skin. EDCs found in soil, air, tap-water, make-up, toys, clothing, textiles, personal care products, food storage containers, carpet and construction materials can cause obesity, insulin resistance or early menopause. They can also activate cancer cells to grow[2].

A December 2021 article by the *San Francisco Chronicle*[3] reported: "Through months of testing, the Center for Environmental Health learned that even small clothing items like socks made for babies, children and adults can be loaded with BPA — up to 31 times the safe limit under California environmental law." The Chronicle continued: "Socks are worn for hours at a time, so it is concerning to find such high levels of BPA, particularly in those made for babies and children." BPA mimics human hormones, the chemical messengers that tell our bodies what to do. Hormones tell a child when to go into puberty. They can tell a woman to go into menopause at age 25. They can tell cancer cells to grow. Hormone-mimicking chemicals can cause nearly every negative health outcome you can think of.

Chemical exposures place higher demands on our system to process and eliminate such chemicals through our liver, lungs, kidneys, intestines and skin. Our body is placed under demand to produce more compounds like glutathione, an antioxidant tripeptide made from three amino acids, in order to protect our cells from damage and to detoxify chemical compounds. Some people may be unable to meet the body's high demands for glutathione. The result is toxic build-up in our cells and cellular damage. Low glutathione levels combined with high EDCs or other chemicals increase oxidative stress in the body, leading to inflammaging and the formation of disease.

Our system is like an air filter with a sensor – in fact, multiple sensors. When the air surrounding the air filter is toxic, the filtration rate and the processing activity of the air filter surge to clean up the dust, fumes, chemicals and mold in the air. All this takes lots of energy, making us tired and exhausted. The accumulation of toxins triggers inflammation, brain fog, hot flashes, sleep disturbances, mood swings, fatigue, digestive issues, joint pain, and blood sugar disturbances. In short: toxins disrupt your capacity to function optimally as a Golden Gate.

As long as this toxic circle continues, inflammation worsens, our mental and emotional muddles, and our physiological systems become chaotic. This ultimately leads to cancer, heart attack, stroke and death. I am struck by the growing number of people in the US with severe chronic complex conditions – many of whom are younger than my patients 20 to 30 years ago. The chronic inflammation and aging that is rampant in so many people I treat is, unfortunately, only the tip of the iceberg as ill-health engulfs our nation at a faster pace than ever before – especially since the pandemic.

Our collective states of physical and mental ill-health result from a multitude of environmental exposures, combined with a lack of self-discipline, morality and spirituality. We are engulfed in a society that creates toxicity at multiple levels because it is based on materialism, greed and lower frequencies of the animalistic nature.

As the population continues to be diagnosed with ever more severe chronic complex diseases, ranging from cancer and heart disease to mysterious neurological conditions, how do we begin to heal our bodies so we can live a more purpose-driven life on our terms, while creating joy and happiness...? It begins with purification and detoxification.

Our Toxic Load

For the past few years, growing evidence suggests a strong link between an individual's exposure to toxins in their environment and in their mind, and the onset of disease and chronic degenerative conditions[4]. The Environmental Protection Agency (EPA) has noted that each toxic substance – which they call a 'toxicant' – at a particular concentration triggers a negative effect on the body.

Environmental toxins have a negative effect on the body even at low doses, and the effect becomes worse with cumulative exposure. For example, a brief exposure to high-frequency radio waves for one to two seconds may have minimal health effects, but frequent radiation exposure or frequent use of microwaves or cell phones accumulates to cause cell damage. One dose of radiation therapy may not cause skin damage, but with every consecutive dose of radiation for a few weeks, the cumulative effect causes more serious symptoms in the region of the treatment like radiation burns and difficulty swallowing, or systemic symptoms like fatigue, immune system changes, or cancer stem cell resistance. Certain symptoms can develop over months, even after radiation therapy has been discontinued[5].

To help our bodies overcome the constant barrage of environmental toxins we are exposed to, we must consciously help our built-in detoxification systems to do their work. Think of it like a vacuum cleaner. If you regularly empty the dust bag and clear blockages in the tubes, the vacuum is able to clean up dust efficiently and it will be less likely to break down. The same is true for our bodies. We must constantly empty our toxic loads, clear blockages, and maintain the health of our cells to slow the aging process and minimize risks of disease formation.

Our toxic load refers to the total accumulated toxins within our system – from our environment, emotions, foods, infections, metals, etc. – that our body has to process. The higher the toxic load, the higher the risk for chronic inflammation, mental illness, cancer, and chronic disease. Toxins cause us to age. The lower we keep our toxic load, the easier it is for our cells to maintain their health and slow down the aging process.

Chronic Health Issues Associated with Environmental Toxic Overload

- Abnormal pregnancy outcomes
- Atherosclerosis
- Brain fog
- Cancer
- Chronic fatigue syndrome
- Chronic immune system depression
- Chronic pain syndrome
- Contact dermatitis
- Fatigue
- Fertility problems
- Fibromyalgia
- Headaches and migraines
- Hormone symptoms and hot flashes
- Increased sensitivity to exogenous exposures, odors or medications
- Joint and body pain
- Kidney dysfunction
- Learning disorders
- Memory loss
- Mineral imbalances (particularly zinc and calcium)
- Mood changes and mood swings
- Multiple chemical sensitivities
- Muscle pain and weakness
- Mast cell conditions
- Non-responsive or recurrent yeast infections
- Numbness and tingling
- Panic attacks
- Parkinson's disease
- Rashes

The goal is to reduce the input of toxins into our cells and tissues and our nervous system, so our body can process and discard any further toxins it comes across. It is like keeping your cup only half full, so that when you are exposed to toxins that are out of your control, your body can still process them and release them with little side effect.

As an integrative naturopathic physician, every day I work on myself to clear imbalances and blockages, and to detoxify and nourish my cells and soul so that I am a hollow reed to allow healing energy to flow through me to my patients. The other day, one of my male patients was shocked to hear I was only a year younger than him. Flatteringly, he thought that I, a 54-year-old woman, was 35 years old. He said to me, "Your skin is not crinkly, your energy is so vibrant, your brain is sharp, and you don't have flabby arms. How is it that you look so young for your age?"

I told him it is because I regularly work at keeping my toxic load down. I have never smoked, consumed alcohol, or used pharmaceutical medications or recreational drugs. I eat organic food, sauna regularly, pray and meditate twice daily, choose the people I hang out with, and so forth. In short, I reduce my toxic load as far as is in my control while optimizing my body's detox systems. All this supports my body in aging slower.

Toxins refer to any substance causing a negative impact on our health. Toxins can be breathed in through our nose and lungs; consumed orally or directly through our veins; absorbed through our skin; produced within our body by metabolic processes, hormones, and internal microbes; or even assimilated into our nervous system through vibrational energetic forces.

Although our bodies are the temple of our precious eternal soul, they house a multitude of toxins – sometimes worse than what we might find on the bottom of the garbage can. Our matrix harbors chemicals, pesticides, hormone by-products, artificial sweeteners, metals, medications, herbicides, and microbes. Our colon inhabits billions of bacteria, mold, yeast, viruses and parasites, plus by-products of hormones, chemicals, inflammation and digested food.

Bacteria, viruses and parasites in the gut or sinuses produce toxins called biotoxins or endotoxins that can travel outside of our gut and sinuses to cause inflammation in joints, in the lining of the heart or lungs, or even in our digestive tract and reproductive organs. Fungi and molds produce toxins called mycotoxins that can invade our nervous system and tissues causing chronic inflammation in the brain, in the blood, in the lungs or in the digestive tract. Some toxins are known as neurotoxins – like from certain forms of mold, viruses, or spirochetes, or from chemicals and metals. They cause inflammation and damage to our nervous system, making us feel brain-fogged, nauseous, moody or dizzy.

Environmental pollutants refer to toxins we are exposed to in our environment through air, water and even food. Household toxins are those usually found in our clothing, furniture, flooring, walls, building materials and cleaning products. Air pollutants include toxins we breathe in like noxious gases. Metal toxins can be found in almost anything, from food, air and water to toys, cookware and our workspaces.

Common Toxins in our Environment

- Arsenic, lead, mercury

- Asbestos

- Chemicals in beauty products (e.g. phthalates, parabens, propylene glycol)

- Dioxins

- Emotional trauma and memories

- Energetic (e.g. cell phones, radiation, people, thoughts)

- Food preservatives, MSG, food coloring, thickeners, gums

- Food/products containing perfluoroalkyl and polyfluoroalkyl (PFAs)

- Gases: ground-level ozone, noxious gasses, cigarette smoke

- Hormone-disrupting chemicals like BPA and phthalates

- Hydrogenated and seed oils

- Metabolic byproducts of the body's own processes or internal microbes

- Metals (e.g. lead, mercury, arsenic, chlorine, fluoride)

- Molds, yeast

- Parasites, fungi, viruses, bacteria

- Particulate matter (e.g. dust, black carbon)

- Pesticides or herbicides (e.g. Atrazine)

- Radon

- Volatile Organic Compounds (e.g. Formaldehyde)

The majority of us women also carry a heavy baggage of emotional toxins: both those created by stress, drama and trauma in our lives, and those that are passed on from one generation to the next. Such emotional toxins can be conscious or subconscious. We hold anger in our liver, resentment in our gallbladder, grief and sadness in our lungs, fear in our kidneys, anxiety in our skin, worry in our spleen and jealousy in every cell of our being.

Be careful of your thoughts and self-talk, especially at bedtime or on waking. When we think negative thoughts at bedtime, we set up our subconscious to produce stress reactions in the body while we sleep, meaning we wake up feeling tired and unrested. Positive thoughts, including saying prayers before bed, and practicing gratitude, are like food for our soul and cells as we sleep. When you wake up and intentionally think positively, you set up your day to attract positivity and healing. The stress reaction or inflammation response for the next day is likely to be lower since you have reduced your mental toxic load before sleep.

Get it Out: Drainage for Healthy Aging

Our skin is the largest excretory organ in the body, with trillions of pores and sweat glands that remove wastes from our inner cells and tissues and help maintain homeostasis. Our skin relates to emotions or fear or anxiety or sadness[6].

Besides the skin, other primary excretory systems, also known as the emunctories, include the liver, lungs, large intestine, kidneys, vagina and emotions[7]. Our intestinal system – a coil of guts that, if stretched out, is at least 30 feet long in most adults – reflects our emotional attachment to things. Hence the expression, "I've got a gut feeling".

Our gallbladder and liver, which are crucial detoxification and drainage organs, process and protect us from toxic and non-toxic chemicals, filter hormones, cleanse our blood, metabolize nutrients and fats while also dealing with viruses, parasites, spirochetes, bacteria, mold, yeast, and anger and resentment.

Our lungs, the organs that bring in oxygen every few seconds to rejuvenate our blood, contain a self-detoxifying system similar to the liver. They use enzyme systems, such as cytochrome p450 and glutathione s-transferase, to break down chemicals and toxins we breathe in[8]. They store sadness and grief.

The kidneys are sensitive organs that take the load off of the lungs and the colon to drain other toxins, such as metals and infections. They are susceptible to blood sugar levels and can get damaged easily. Kidneys house fear, according to Eastern medicine.

Monthly excretion of menstrual flow through the vagina, and the natural vaginal excretions, play a vital role in maintaining women's health and fertility. Without this drainage, congestion builds up leading to infections and disease. Intimate relationships are housed in this area and when there are past or current relationship stressors, vaginal drainage may be impeded leading to bloating, pelvic congestion, vaginal dryness and other pelvic disorders.

Keeping our primary emunctories open, to allow for continual drainage and removal of waste and toxins, helps maintain good health while reducing the toxic burden in our cells. When these primary emunctories become overloaded or blocked, and the secondary emunctories become further stressed, this triggers free radical formation, cellular damage and the development of symptoms. Over time, this leads to the formation of disease.

For example, when you are constipated either emotionally or physically, the body cannot drain out heavy metals, chemicals or infections. The skin may present with acne or eczema, or the lungs may become asthmatic. If chronic constipation persists over decades, colon cancer or lung cancer can form. Practicing a lifestyle that continues to maintain open emunctories helps reduce chronic disease and also helps you feel free and open to the challenges life may bring you.

Our secondary emunctories include the skin, muscles, joints, bones, lymphatic system, mucous membranes and emotions. The lymphatic system, an open system consisting of a mesh of lymphatic vessels, nodes, organs and lymphoid tissue, sweeps toxins from tissues and dumps them into the blood to be processed and discarded through the primacy emunctories. The lymphatic system plays an important role in immune defense and calibrates the body fluid, electrolytes and nutrients while guarding the body from foreign invasion. The glymphatic system comprised of glial cells is responsible for waste clearance of the central nervous system in the brain[9]. Breast tissue contains three layers of lymphatic tissue, and the head and neck – including the gums and teeth – contain a third of all the lymph nodes in the body[10].

This means that when infections and toxins harbor in the mouth, there is a very high chance it will impact disease processes in the rest of the body. When the lymphatic system is burdened by infections, metals or mold toxins, its flow slows. Then congestion builds and, over time, inflammation and cancer may ensue. Hence, a congested lymphatic system as found in periodontal disease is clearly related to increased inflammation markers, heart disease[11], kidney disease[12] and breast cancer[13]. There is a significant link between oral health and breast cancer – particularly in post-menopausal women[14]. I find the lymphatic system holds stubbornness, obstinacy and stagnation. Emotions such as anger, grief or fear that are stuck, mainly as a defense mechanism, can cause the lymphatic system and the immune system to weaken[15]. Surgical scars often create physical and energetic blockages in the lymphatic flow.

Different daily techniques to assist drainage, especially of the lymphatic system, help reduce toxic build-up. Homeopathic drainage remedies, neural therapy injections to break up scars, lymphatic massage, dry brushing and aerobic exercise, including walking, offer easy support for lymphatic movement and drainage.

While the lymphatic system drains physical toxins, the most important system for emotional detoxification and drainage is our soul. Continually working on the drainage of the emotions and soul through meditation and prayer, practicing virtues, and unconditional acts of service, helps keep our soul aligned with our individual and collective meaningful purpose. Such practices keep us feeling elevated, elated and clear.

Detox or Depurate?

The term "detoxification" or "detox" has found its place in many fad diets, recipes, marketing schemes, websites, blogs, spas, integrative medical practices and books. The "detox diet", "detox yoga", and "detox facial" are examples of the marketing used to lure patients to purchase products that may or may not reduce the body's toxic load.

The use of the word "detox" or "detoxification" in these cases is incorrect. The word "depurate" or "depuration" is a better word choice. "Depuration" is a broader term referring to purification of the mind, body and spirit. It implies purifying or cleansing all our cells and organs, including our thoughts and emotions. When we do yoga, we are not only optimizing the biochemical detoxification of the liver, we are also purifying ourselves of physical, emotional and energetic toxins. We are depurating.

"Detoxification" refers specifically to the biochemical process that occurs in the liver and colon to rid the body of toxic chemicals and hormones. Detoxification uses three phases, each requiring certain nutrients to optimize liver, colon and kidney functions to rid the body of chemicals and toxins.

Phase I detoxification involves using oxygen to make toxic compounds, chemicals and hormones more water-soluble in the liver, using the cytochrome P450 enzyme system. Phase I is like emptying out the closet. The process requires B-vitamins, amino acids, magnesium, iron, minerals, glutathione and bioflavonoids. Caffeine, alcohol and environmental toxins activate Phase I while soy, garlic, and grapefruit juice inhibit it. Carotenoids found in carrots and colored veggies, alongside vitamin C, vitamin E, copper, manganese, zinc and coenzyme Q10, protect cells from being damaged by overactivation of Phase I[16].

Phase II detox, masterfully regulated by the Nrf2 gene, involves neutralizing toxins and making them more water-soluble. I like to think of Phase II as the process of packaging toxins into garbage bags to be eliminated later through the bowels or urine. This particular stage requires glutathione and amino acids such as cysteine, glycine, glutamine, and taurine. Co-factors such as B-vitamins, NAC (N-acetylcysteine) and methionine are also needed for Phase II. Sulfur-rich foods like garlic, eggs, onions and cruciferous veggies, as well as methyl donors like TMG (trimethylglycine), further support Phase II detoxification[17].

Phase II is induced by Nrf2 activators like berberine, green tea extract, quercetin, curcumin, milk thistle, genistein from soy and resveratrol, as well as sulforaphane foods from the broccoli family of veggies. Furthermore, fermented foods, like sauerkraut and tempeh, and drinks, like kefir, provide small electrochemicals called alkyl catechols, which also activate Nrf2 to trigger Phase II detoxification.

The final elimination stage of detoxification, Phase III, involves getting the garbage bags out of the house. In the case of our bodies, this means pumping the neutralized substances out of liver cells into bile to be eliminated through the colon, or out of kidney cells into urine. Phase III is referred to as the transporter phase as the garbage bags are transported out to the dumpster by the garbage truck. This phase requires fiber, a healthy microbiome, L-glutamine, and calcium d-glucarate for optimum function. Herbal extracts like artichoke leaf extract, dandelion root extract, black radish, and yellow dock root, plus adequate water intake, and an alkaline diet, can also further support this final phase[18].

In order to prevent the house from getting stinky during detoxification, and to clean up the dusty remnants left behind during the elimination process, nutrients such as vitamins A, C, E, selenium, zinc, copper, CoQ10 and bioflavonoids are necessary. Detoxifying the body can help eliminate toxins, hormones, microbes, metals and metabolic wastes that create inflammation, interfere with optimal cellular function and cause aging. Detoxification is therefore an important biochemical process, especially in the liver and intestines. In functional naturopathic medicine, we combine biochemical detoxification with removing and correcting the underlying causes of metabolic, nutritional and biochemical imbalances within each patient.

Energetically, detoxifying allows for associated stuck emotions – like anger and resentment in the liver or emotional and mental attachments in the colon – to be released as physical toxins are eliminated. Regular detoxifying helps us clear the physical and emotional barriers to accessing our spiritual capacities.

Why Depurate?

Depuration is vital to our wellbeing. It clears our minds, helping us get rid of brain fog, confusion and stagnant thinking. It clears our physical tissues to reduce pain in joints and muscles and improve digestive health. Depuration improves our memory and intellect and gives us a stronger capacity to reflect and meditate, through which we discover the hidden mysteries of the world. It opens the doorway to health and wellness physically, mentally, emotionally and spiritually.

Our body is naturally equipped to depurate. We sweat to release impurities and defecate to expel toxins in the colon and intestines. We exhale to clean our blood and lungs of toxic carbon dioxide. We urinate to clean our kidneys and the blood. Optimizing these depuration systems – sweating, respiration, defecation, and urination – helps us depurate naturally, thereby improving our health and our capacity to age youthfully. See Appendix A for a full list of foods that support depuration and detoxification, and a list of easy ways to support depuration. Further depuration tips are available at GoldenGateBook.com/resources.

We have also been given the tools to depurate our emotions. The purification of our emotions occurs naturally through crying, talking, singing, screaming, laughter and movement such as dancing, running and walking. Using these depuration systems regularly helps clean our emotions and the baggage we often carry. We mentally depurate through our abilities of writing, reading, drawing, imagining, visualizing, processing, meditating, and understanding. Regular mindful practice of these depuration processes strengthens and clears our minds and mental function, allowing us to stay focused and grounded.

The act of prayer and meditation purifies our spirit. The more we meditate and pray, the stronger our connection to our spirit and the easier the road to health and wellness. Meditation and prayer allow us to discover the hidden mysteries and treasures within the universe. Meditation opens access to universal knowledge of the past, present and the future. Therefore, meditation and prayer are forms of depuration for our soul.

Let It Go!

As crazy as it may sound, most of us women have a hard time letting go of toxins, especially emotional ones. In many cases, our cells, tissues and organs and, above all, our emotional memory develop a hoarding behavior. We hoard infections, chemicals, metals, pesticides, sugars and, of course, stress and emotions – to name only a few. And most women hoard the heaviest baggage of them all: the baggage of drama, trauma and emotions.

Our emotional baggage is like a security blanket. We have carried it so carefully for years, added to it almost daily, and become deeply attached to it. Our emotional luggage is so personal and, at times, so heavy it weighs us down, bringing down with it our energy, our mental outlook, our relationships, and our zest for life.

In some ways, our attachment to these toxic emotions has become our trademark. We have formed mechanisms and unconsciously mutated some of our genes to reduce our ability to depurate them and to make ourselves unknowingly even more toxic. Then we unknowingly pass these genetic mutations to our children… and they learn to pack all of our toxins as well as their own.

Think about how you may carry some of your mom's emotional baggage or her unresolved emotions. Many of us do this starting from childhood. We want to save our parents from their misery, so we carry their stuff thinking we are saving them. Instead, we create lifelong chronic illness for ourselves and steal the opportunity from our parents for their growth. And as we grow into adulthood, we do the same for our partners.

Why do we do this to ourselves? Why don't we just let go? We would be so much happier and satisfied with our lives if we could learn from men and let it go. What is keeping us from cleansing these toxic memories and emotions?

What many of us don't realize is that the same powerful capacity to mutate our genes to something negative also has the capacity to transform our genes to something more positive. This is the power of epigenetics.

For instance, research is beginning to show how we can use our thoughts, emotions and meditation to create positive processes within our cells. In fact, such practices can potentially shift our gene expression and our DNA methylation profile, slow aging by increasing telomere length[19] (a marker of aging), improve oxygen flow, reduce stress and enhance DNA repair[20]. Just as we can unconsciously reduce our detoxification and immune systems, disrupt our microbiome and increase the oxidative stress in our cells, we also can enhance our detoxification and methylation processes, boost our immune function, improve our microbiome and decrease our oxidative stress by practicing a conscious, elevated lifestyle. We consciously can change our cellular milieu.

Practicing mindful meditation has been shown to reduce symptoms of Long-COVID and post-viral conditions such as myalgic encephalomyelitis (ME) and post-viral fatigue[21]. It can also improve neuroplasticity in major depression[22]. Conscious eating, thinking, exercising and, most importantly, conscious meditation, prayer and emotional clearing become the hallmark for continual detoxification, regeneration, and optimization of our physical, mental and emotional health. Putting it all together, I call it practicing being a "conscious being".

We are spiritual beings journeying this world in a physical realm, and so when we become aware of our blockages, the process of awareness itself causes a release. We hold on to our toxins as if we would not survive without them. Yet in reality we would be healthier, happier and age more youthfully if we got rid of all the baggage – the toxic emotions, infections, chemicals, pollutants and metals – that create a veil covering our soul so our soul can fully express itself.

Case Study: Releasing Emotional Trauma

A 33-year-old mother of a three-year-old daughter came to me with extreme muscle and generalized body pain, dizziness, fainting spells, weakness and low stamina.

She began her treatment by reducing toxic exposures. Then she learnt how to replenish and nourish herself, both emotionally and physically. Once she had been nourished with food, nutrients and self-compassion she was ready to release.

We supported her emunctories and depuration systems and then identified and treated the chronic infections she was harboring. We worked with her to balance her hormones and stress response. But some of her pains and symptoms did not shift until we helped her identify and release the associated emotional trauma she had suffered at three years of age when she was abandoned by her mother. Her father remarried a woman who did not pay much attention to her as a child either. She felt abandoned by both parents and alone.

As we released her emotional childhood pain using a combination of techniques like EMDR, ND Square™, brain-spotting and family constellation work, her pain and physical symptoms significantly reduced. She then worked on restoring the empty sensation with love, honor and gratitude for her mother and father.

Her pain resolved. She no longer experiences fainting spells, weakness or body pain episodes. She now exhibits vitality, gratitude and joy and is back at work and taking care of her daughter.

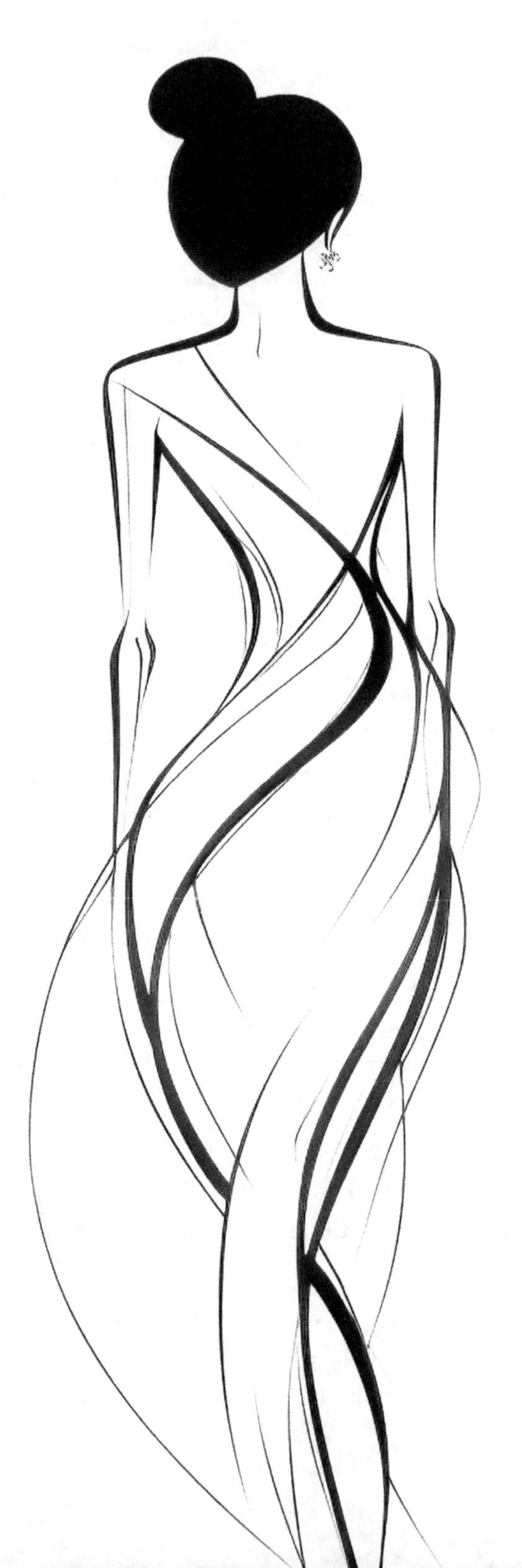

Chapter 11

Your
Gut
Feeling

"For every part
of the universe
is connected with every
other by ties that are
very powerful and admit
no imbalance,
nor any slackening..."

'Abdu'l-Bahá

The human body is a remarkable and intricately interconnected system, where various organs and processes work in harmony to maintain optimal health. Among the many components that contribute to this intricate balance, the gut stands out as a vital hub of activity with profound implications for the wellbeing of the entire body, including the brain.

Most of us understand the gut to be the place where food is broken down, digested, and absorbed. But in the last couple of decades, we have discovered that the gut is much more than just a churning machine for food. Beyond its role in assimilating, absorbing and digesting nutrients, the gut wields a considerable influence over a wide range of bodily functions including immune responses, hormone regulation, nervous system reactions and even mental health. The gut is the crossroads where the nervous system, immune system, hormonal system, digestion and emotional systems meet, communicate and relay information to the rest of the body, including the brain. For this vital work connecting the systems that keep our bodies ticking over as they should, I often refer to the gut as "the grand central station" or "the second brain".

The gut houses and regulates emotions and neurotransmitters (including chemicals involved with anxiety and depression), it metabolizes hormones, and it protects us from invasive infections like the COVID-19 virus, colds and flus, as well as chronic infections such as parasites and tick-borne diseases. Furthermore, disease often starts in the gut, decades before it shows up in the nervous system. For instance, scientists find Lewy bodies in the gut several years before they find them in the brain of Parkinson's patients[1]. And did you know your gut is also involved in decision-making? All this information gets communicated to the brain through a variety of different pathways.

The Magic of the Microbiome

The majority of the gut's functions are performed by the bacteria in your gut, called the gut microbiota, which make up the gut microbiome. To give you an idea of the importance of this forgotten 'metabolic organ', the microbiome weighs between two and six pounds and contains around 100 trillion gut bacteria from more than 1,000 different species[2].

By acting as a signaling network, the microbiome influences the functions of our brain, lungs, heart, kidneys and liver. Any disruption in the microbiome may contribute to disease progression of all kinds, including mood disorders. That's right: these 100 trillion gut bacteria living in your intestines produce, regulate, and transport chemicals that make you happy, anxious or sad. There are ten times more gut bacteria in our bodies than human cells, and 100 times more bacteria genetic material than human genes.

Changes in the microbiome can trigger inflammation or pain, or reduce inflammation and act as a sedative. Your gut bacteria process your hormones and regulate hormone metabolism. For instance, they secrete β-glucuronidase to reduce circulating levels of estrogen. This is known as the estrogen-gut microbiome axis. When it malfunctions, it is linked to the development of a range of conditions such as obesity, metabolic syndrome, cancer, endometrial hyperplasia, endometriosis, polycystic ovary syndrome, infertility and cardiovascular disease[3].

Furthermore, the gut bacteria play an intricate role in regulating bone health, by interacting with the parathyroid hormone[4]. They also play a vital role in regulating our immune system. A thriving gut microbiota bolsters the body's defense mechanisms, helping to recognize and eliminate pathogens. Moreover, an imbalanced gut microbiome has been implicated in autoimmune conditions, allergies, and chronic inflammatory diseases. Nurturing gut health is therefore a cornerstone of a resilient immune system and comprehensive wellbeing.

In fact, approximately 70-80% of the immune system exists in the gut[5]. The gut's microbiome protects us from infections. When the microbiome becomes imbalanced or low in bacteria diversity, inflammation increases as proinflammatory cytokines (chemicals released by immune cells) are released. This compromises immune-surveillance and alters immune cell profiles, increasing our risk of cancer and making us more susceptible to infections.

When a patient is infected with COVID-19 (correctly called the SARS-CoV-2 virus), we observe disturbances in the gut microbiome, with loss of bacteria diversity, an increase in pathogenic bacteria, and activation of inflammation[6]. Decreased diversity poses a risk for increased gut inflammation, and often leads to wider systemic inflammation around the body (including the lungs through the gut-lung axis) and the onset of disease. Diabetics, for instance, often have an imbalanced gut microbiome with low diversity, resulting in lowered immune function[7]. Hence, during the pandemic, diabetics were at a higher risk of complications and death from the COVID-19 virus[8].

Opportunistic bacteria, fungi, and viruses increase as a result of the weakened gut microbiome network during COVID-19 infection. This increases the growth of infections like candidiasis (yeast overgrowth). In patients with Long-COVID, these changes in the microbiome continue for months after the acute infection[9]. A weakened microbiome and low gut bacteria diversity also play a major role in the development and progression of autoimmune disease, chronic infections, cancer and metabolic conditions. Strengthening the microbiome through fasting and a low-carb diet that is high in plants and healthy fats can improve the outcome of treatment for cancer patients and slow tumor progression[10].

Each one of us has a unique microbiome that we inherited from our mother. Its health depends on our environment, stress levels and emotions, exercise, and the food we eat. Babies born naturally through the vaginal canal become inoculated with the mother's microbiome. Those born by C-section often do not have the initial microbiome inoculation and may have more immune conditions in the first months of their life because of lowered bacterial diversity[11]. It takes at least three years for children to build their gut microbiota[12]. Thus, a healthy plant-based, low processed diet during those initial three years of life sets up the child for lifelong health[13]. And mothers-to-be maintaining a healthy microbiome leads to healthier babies being born.

The Gut-Brain Axis

The microbes in the gut regulate the production, transportation, and functioning of neurotransmitters (the neurochemicals involved with mood). When the gut ecosystem falls out of balance, our mood and behavior change, depression and anxiety worsen, and our memory diminishes. Thanks to the vital role our gut plays in regulating our brain function, the latest medical studies on mood and behavior disorders focus on the gut microbiome.

Mounting evidence now supports the theory that disruption of the microbiome and low gut bacteria diversity increases the risk of developing neurodegenerative or neuroinflammatory conditions such as dementia, epilepsy, autism, Alzheimer's or Parkinson's[14]. Patients with these conditions have a lower diversity of gut bacteria, and the balance is skewed towards higher amounts of pathogenic bacteria (such as Escherichia coli/Shigella, Bacteroides) and lower levels of beneficial bacteria (such as Eubacterium Rectale and Bifidobacterium)[15].

Antibiotics literally destroy the microbiota diversity. In the very young, before age three, and the older population, the diminished gut microbiota diversity poses risks for neuroinflammation. However, modulating the gut microbiota[16] through a Mediterranean diet[17,18], probiotics, cultured foods[19] and turmeric extract (curcumin)[20,21] may potentially slow such neurodegenerative and neuroinflammatory conditions.

The communication between the brain, gut and microbiome is complex and works in both directions. This means that what we perceive and think can affect the gut microbiome, our hormones, and our inflammation. Conversely, the presence of certain bacteria in the gut can impact brain function, our thoughts and our memory[22]. Because the gut-brain connection also involves the immune system and the endocrine (hormone) system, the microbiome gut health influences our immune function and hormones. However, our hormone system and the status of our immune system can also impact the microbiome, our gut and brain health.

These communications take place through our vagus nerve (the most important nerve in the body as it innervates almost every organ) and the nerves in the gut (known as the enteric nerves). Inflammation in the brain occurs when chemicals known as endotoxins and lipopolysaccharides are released by the gut bacteria and travel in the blood to the brain, activating an immune response in the brain that leads to inflammation.

Most of us experience this brain inflammation as 'brain fog', which feels like one's thinking is cloudy or the brain feels heavy. Many people with COVID-19 experienced brain fog, which results from the immune reaction in the brain in response to the disruption of the gut microbiome during the illness[23].

Some may have very light symptoms of the COVID-19 virus in the initial phases of the infection, but may go on to experience the brain fog, memory issues, and brain fatigue weeks later. This condition is categorized as Long-COVID or post-COVID syndrome and it involves the disturbed microbiome[24]. Dysregulated hormones, resulting from disruption in the microbiome during ovulation, pre-menstruation or perimenopause, may also cause brain fog, anxiety and depression[25].

Depression and anxiety have also worsened since the pandemic. The gut microbiome can produce neurotransmitters, or activate the release of neurotransmitters, in response to emotional stress and an infection, such as the spike proteins of the COVID-19 virus found in the gut. Within milliseconds, the chemicals released in response to the virus travel to the brain through the vagus nerve and trigger an inflammatory response in the brain. Brain fog, memory issues and cognitive issues result. Thus, emotional trauma and its related stress response can literally change the microbiome and make you more susceptible to getting COVID-19 or experiencing Long-COVID neuroinflammation symptoms, like brain fog and cognitive dysfunction.

The Estrogen–Gut Link

One of the most important links in the body is the gut-estrogen connection: the estrobolome[26]. The estrobolome consists of a collection of bacteria in the gut that support estrogen metabolism and metabolize and modulate the estrogens circulating in the blood. When healthy levels of the estrobolome are present, an enzyme known as β-glucuronidase, which activates estrogens into their active form, is balanced and relatively low. Estrogens are therefore eliminated through the colon and prevented from re-circulating back into the bloodstream.

When there is bacterial imbalance, such as in dysbiosis, gram-negative bacteria prevail in the estrobolome. This produces higher levels of β-glucuronidase, which causes estrogens to recirculate back into the bloodstream through the gut wall[27]. Higher levels of β-glucuronidase in the gut have been associated with an increased risk of breast cancer, obesity, lowered libido and depression. Estrogens reabsorbed into the blood through the gut lining increase toxicity, estrogen dominance and cell inflammation, further stressing the liver and the detoxification system. These recirculating estrogens also activate hormone-related cancer growth.

Several factors influence a healthy estrobolome and lower levels of β-glucuronidase, including genetics, diet and nutrition, perceived stress, medications like antibiotics, alcohol intake, and environmental exposures. Furthermore, a bi-directional relationship exists between the estrobolome and estrogens, meaning when toxic estrogens are consumed or metabolic conditions such as insulin resistance exist, the estrobolome also gets disturbed[28].

To improve the estrobolome and reduce the bacteria that produce β-glucuronidase, a plant-based diet high in fiber, cruciferous vegetables, fermented foods, and prebiotic foods like artichoke, garlic, dandelion greens, chicory root, leeks and asparagus can be highly supportive[29]. Reducing overall exposure to toxins – especially man-made chemicals that act like estrogens called xenoestrogens (found in plastics, hair spray and herbicides, for instance) and improving insulin resistance and metabolic concerns also supports a healthy estrobolome[30,31]. Taking calcium d-glucarate supplements helps bind β-glucuronidase enzyme, thereby reducing recirculating estrogens[32].

The Importance of Oral Health

The microbiome in our mouth plays a crucial role in maintaining both oral and overall health, influencing functions from digestion and immune response to disease prevention. Imbalances in the mouth microbiome can elevate the risk of conditions such as dental caries, gum disease and even systemic diseases like cardiovascular disorders and cancer[33].

Whatever is in our mouth, we swallow into our gut, affecting the gut microbiota. The mouth houses over 700 different species of bacteria. These bacteria can hide inside root canals, in gingival sulcus, in the teeth, the gums, the inner cheek, the hard palate, tongue, tonsils and soft palate.

Our diet and oral hygiene habits impact oral health. For example, diets high in processed foods and sugars have a negative impact on the oral microbiome, while a Mediterranean diet rich in omega 3 fatty acids, fermented foods, whole foods, and fruit and vegetables has a positive impact on the health of the oral microbiome[34]. A February 2023 study looking at over 5,651 patients over the age of 40 found that a healthy plant-based diet is associated with reduced risks of periodontal disease and improved oral microbiome[35].

Modern technology gives researchers the tools to identify the relationship between poor oral microbiome and the presence of systemic diseases such as Alzheimer's[36], heart disease[37], cancer[38], obesity[39], rheumatoid arthritis[40], lung conditions[41] and liver conditions such as NASH (non-alcoholic liver disease)[42]. Periodontal disease has even been linked to arthritis (joint pain)[43].

Periodontal disease and stealth infections in the mouth, especially within root canals, around titanium dental implants or in areas of dental extractions (called cavitations), have been linked to breast cancer and the severity of other types of cancers[44,45]. In fact, a December 2023 study found that periodontal disease affects the initiation and development of breast cancer involving micro-organisms and inflammation[46]. In another study, researchers hypothesized that the health status of the oral microbiome and the presence of periodontal disease are such strong indicators that they may be used as a non-invasive biomarker for cancer risk in the future[47].

The health of your mouth, gums and teeth may be the initiator of many other conditions, too. Every patient I have treated for neurological conditions like dementia, Alzheimer's, Parkinson's, multiple sclerosis and glioblastoma have always had major dental concerns, such as high amounts of old leaky mercury amalgams, untreated stealth dental infections and severe oral dysbiosis.

Case Study: How Are Your Teeth?

My father suffered from bad teeth for most of his adult years. He had titanium dental implants, gold crowns, several extractions, and silver amalgams. His oral microbiome was definitely not healthy and his local dentists did not know how to correct it.

He suffered debilitating arthritis of his knee, which I believe was a result of the chronic inflammation in his mouth stressing his lymphatic and immune system. His chronic arthritis was perhaps linked to the dysbiosis of his mouth and teeth filled with toxic metals. Later on, he sadly developed colon cancer on the same side as his dental concerns and his arthritic knee.

So, you see how dental toxicities probably led to chronic inflammation in the knees and, finally, resulted in colon cancer on the same side of the body. Every time he ate or drank, he was swallowing those same bacteria and toxic metals down to the intestines. As his body tried to clear the toxicity through the bowels, it led to further dysbiosis and toxic overload in his colon. His body tried to correct it for a long time and finally gave up by creating a tumor. Do you now see how the body is all connected?

Sadly, my father's dental care was provided by 'old-fashioned' dentists with little knowledge of the whole-body connection to the teeth. Luckily, we now have biological dentists who safely remove silver amalgams, address the oral microbiome, and use ceramic or zirconium implants rather than titanium implants. They understand the connection between the health of the teeth, gums, jawbones and the rest of the body, and vice versa. A healthy mouth supports a healthy gut microbiome – and therefore, a healthy mind, hormones and body.

Each cancer patient I have worked with in the last 28 years has also had some type of oral dysbiosis or untreated periodontal disease caused by amalgams, or the presence of at least two different dental metals in the mouth, or titanium dental implants, infected root canals, and/or unhealthy oral care. I always refer my chronically ill patients to a biological dentist who addresses these concerns and uses compatible dental materials while testing patients for oral dysbiosis.

Regulation thermometry, a computerized system using an infrared thermometer to detect heat patterns and physiological dysfunction, provides an easy evaluation of the hidden inflammation in the teeth/jaw region and associated lymphatic system function. The heat patterns identified can indicate hidden infections, metal toxicity or reduced lymphatic drainage linked to autonomic nervous system dysfunction and organ stress in the rest of the body. It can pick up problems that dental X-rays may miss. This assessment helps me identify when to refer patients to dentists for re-evaluation of a possible important link between their mouth and their body condition.

I have found baking soda to be the simplest and most effective way to clean teeth non-abrasively and to maintain a healthy oral microbiome. It is significantly better than most toothpastes in cleaning teeth and gums and normalizing mouth acidity, and it is definitely less toxic than typical brand toothpaste. Incidentally, most toothpaste and mouthwashes on the market actually disrupt the oral microbiome and the pH, setting us up for not only dental and gum issues but also chronic health problems. The advantages of using baking soda as toothpaste is that it reduces plaque and gingivitis, it can reduce bacteria, it whitens teeth, it provides a fluoride-free option and it is inexpensive.

How to make homemade baking soda toothpaste

You'll need:

- a toothbrush

- a small bowl or shot glass

- baking soda

- Optional essential oil (peppermint oil, orange essence oil, lemon or lime essential oil, or bergamot oil)

- Filtered or distilled water

Instructions:

- First, mix equal parts baking soda and filtered water in a small bowl until you've created a paste. Add in a couple of drops of the essential oil of your choice.

- Dip your toothbrush into the soda mix and brush in gentle circles, making sure you cover each tooth thoroughly with the paste. Massage your gums with your toothbrush.

- Keep brushing for around a minute. When you're done, spit out the baking soda and rinse until your teeth are grit-free and shiny.

Is Your Brain on Fire?

Our sinuses play a crucial role in our overall health by helping to filter, humidify and regulate the air we breathe, while contributing to the resonance of our voice and protecting our brain and eyes. Our sinuses are the closed hollow caves in our face, and are lined with mucous membranes like our mouth and gut. Technically, they are part of the respiratory tract, but I also see them as part of the alimentary tract. Anything we inhale travels through the sinuses, which join the mouth at the back of the throat, can potentially go down our windpipe to our lungs or enter our digestive tract through the esophagus.

The olfactory nerve, the smell nerve, innervates the main sinuses (maxillary sinuses) in our face and directly links to our brain. This means anything we breathe in or smell can travel directly into the brain without any surveillance. That's why toxic fumes, molds, perfumes and smoke can give us headaches and brain fog when we smell them because they cause brain inflammation. I always purchase less toxic, formaldehyde-free nail polish. Less toxic nail polish may not last as long, but it saves my brain from overload.

One time, as I walked up the stairs to my teenage daughters' bedroom, I could smell toxic fumes. Immediately, I got nauseous with a forehead headache – a sign of liver distress. I couldn't help but burst out in anger – a liver emotion. The three of them were sitting there innocently painting their nails with nail polish they had acquired from a friend. The fumes from those tiny bottles were so intense that just the tiny amount of chemical particles hitting my olfactory nerve caused an immediate inflammatory reaction in my brain, giving me a headache and nausea and making me uncontrollably emotionally reactive.

From then on, my girls learnt that commercial nail polish contains very toxic chemicals, namely phthalates, formaldehyde and toluene, which disrupt hormones, induce inflammation of the nervous system and overload the liver. They can literally cause you to feel crazy. That's also why you may feel unlike yourself – crazy at times – when you are premenstrual, ovulating or perimenopausal: the endocrine disrupters you have been exposed during the month cause your brain to be on fire as hormones peak during these times of the month[48].

This same type of reaction may also be caused by mold and mycotoxins (toxins from mold), by smoke, radon, and many other chemicals we are not even aware we are smelling. Many toxins we breathe in are odorless and we have no idea we are breathing them in. Instead, we wonder why we are getting frustrated or depressed, or wonder why our children are acting out, having trouble concentrating, experiencing stomach pains, or being diagnosed with ADHD.

Because such substances we smell are toxic to the nervous system, the immune system alerts the body through inflammation in the brain[49]. Nervous system symptoms, like depression, anxiety, brain fog, headache and anger are the result of this brain inflammation signaling danger. Pro-inflammatory chemicals, called cytokines, are released by the immune system in the brain to eliminate the invaders entering the nervous system as quickly as possible. Our mental, emotional and physical symptoms are the result of the immune sirens and first responders responding to danger by trying to shut down the fire and clean up the toxicity. Literally, the brain is on fire with inflammation. It is actually known as 'brain on fire'[50], as depicted by Calahan in her 2012 book, *Brain on Fire: My Month of Madness*. Headaches, anger, brain fog, focus issues, seizures, mood changes and memory issues are signs of your brain's immune reaction to the invader – signs your brain is on fire.

Our environment – what we inhale, smell, and are exposed to – can be either an invader or a healer. By accessing the brain through the nose, we can inhale essential oils, like lavender or lemon balm oil, to calm the nervous system, relieving depression, brain fog, and stomach aches. Glutathione, a super antioxidant, may be nebulized through the nose to the brain to modulate brain and sinus inflammation[51] and detox the brain[52].

Since the sinuses are a closed cavity with limited drainage, they often house persistent infections like mold, yeast, bacteria or biofilm (similar to dental plaques where bacteria are housed) long-term. This can lead to chronic sinus inflammation, post-nasal drip and sinus allergies, as well as systemic symptoms like fatigue, brain fog, and digestive issues. The chronic inflammatory response to persisting infections and their associated toxins stresses the lymphatic and the digestive systems. Our lymphatic system cleans out tissues and moves byproducts of infections into the blood to be eliminated through the emunctories, organs of elimination. When sinuses are chronically inflamed, the whole body's lymphatic system becomes constantly overloaded, making you feel tired, bloated, in pain and stressed.

In chronically ill or chronically fatigued women, I often find chronic infection of sinuses with antibiotic-resistant staph infections (known either as MRCoNS[53,54] or MRSA). Chronic dental infections from dental implants[55] can also invade the sinuses and cause chronic infections in the sinuses which can lead to whole-body illness, fatigue or brain fog.

In many instances, the microbiota of the sinus cavities may therefore be as important to evaluate as the microbiota of the gut. In my chronically ill female patients who are not improving as much as I expect them to, I usually order a bacterial, fungal, and biofilm culture of the sinus cavities to evaluate the microbiota and chronic infections. Additionally, I refer them to a biological dentist for a comprehensive dental and jaw evaluation and to an ENT (head and nose) specialist to check no other pathology exists.

The Power of the Pelvis

Our pelvis is the center of our life force, our 'dan tian', or our 'sea of energy' as in Asian martial arts. Formed from three bones, our pelvis is the largest bowl in the body housing three different organ systems: the bladder, the sigmoid/rectum section of the colon and our reproductive organs. The pelvic floor consists of 26 muscles. We collect energy associated with relationships, fertility, security, safety and power in the pelvis. The pelvis is also associated with intuition, creative expression and, of course, sexual intimacy, relationships and birthing.

Pelvic health is crucial for women as untreated chronic pelvic pain can potentially worsen underlying conditions, leading to a cascade of negative health effects. One in seven women in the US suffers from chronic pelvic pain, which is defined as pelvic pain experienced longer than three months[56]. It is often associated with irritable bowel syndrome, depression and/or pelvic inflammatory syndrome. Chronic pelvic pain has recently been identified to be complex and caused by multiple factors, requiring a multidisciplinary approach to its treatment. But Western medicine mainly offers pain medications and/or surgery as treatment, and the underlying root causes continue to be dismissed.

Acupuncture, manual therapy, manipulation, auricular therapy and light therapy have been recently studied to help with pelvic pain[57]. Alongside these techniques, I also employ neural therapy, homeopathy and somatic work to ease chronic pelvic pain. The goal is not to suppress the pain but to identify the root causes – and one of the major causes of chronic pelvic pain is suppressed emotions.

In the pelvis, we tend to house our emotions and the energy of our relationships, old and new. We carry the energy of our first love, past abusive relationships, miscarriages, abortions, our wounds and our secrets. In his bestselling book *The Body Keeps the Score*, psychiatrist Bessel van der Kolk examines how trauma is held in the memory of our somatic nervous system and is then often expressed as a biological response. I have seen how unresolved suppressed emotions can manifest in physical symptoms. For example, patients who have suffered sexual abuse or a traumatic birth later develop uterine fibroids, chronic pelvic pain or pelvic tumors. Our nervous system responds to trauma through tightening, pain, freezing, numbing and holding.

Homeopathy, somatic emotional release work, brain-spotting, and many other techniques help resolve the connection between the unresolved emotion and the physical body. Using a technique I created called ND Square™, my work shifts the link between the autonomic nervous system, its fight-and-flight response, the physical symptoms and pain, the associated emotions, and the somatic cellular memory. Many women carry unresolved trauma from past generations within the pelvis. When we identify and acknowledge these deep-seeded emotions and honor, thank and pray for the ancestor who suffered the original trauma, chronic pain often resolves.

Homeopathic medicines, such as potentized estrogen, can also be helpful in reducing pelvic pain, depression, anxiety and emotions resulting from trauma[58]. Energy exercises like Qi Gong, which focus on the dan tian, can also help. In a double-blind, placebo-controlled clinical trial[59] of 50 women aged 18-45, homeopathic estrogen significantly reduced symptoms of pelvic pain, cyclical urinary pain, cyclical bowel pain, depression and anxiety in women suffering from endometriosis. In another two-year study[60], 46% of 128 women who were treated with homeopathy saw their menstrual cramps improve by more than 50%.

For the first four years of my marriage, despite not using birth control, I did not get pregnant until I began working on my dan tian. Tai Chi exercises focusing on the dan tian increase physiological and energetic circulation to the pelvic bowl. As I released old energy, stagnation resolved and healthy energy and circulation moved into my pelvis. Within a couple of months of starting Tai Chi I became pregnant with my first child.

Listen to Your Gut Feeling

As we have now seen, the human body is an intricately interconnected system, a complex dance of bodily functions that work in harmony to maintain optimal health. In this complex dance, the gut emerges as a central orchestrator, woven into the fabric of our wellbeing.

The remarkable interplay between the gut and the brain, extending its influence to systemic health and immune resilience, reinforces the importance of nurturing gut health. As we embark on a journey to prioritize our wellbeing, the importance of the gut becomes increasingly evident, encouraging us to foster a harmonious gut-brain connection. Looking after our oral, sinus and pelvic health is key too, to support the gut's vital work.

From my own experience treating thousands of women, backed by latest research, it is evident how important the efficient function of the gut microbiota and microbiome is on our health, and how great an impact it has on the health of future generations. The microbiome and microbiota diversity that our babies inherit from us at birth, and the diet we feed them, potentially determines their long-term health risks and the health of generations to come.

An article in Medical News Today[61] sums up the future of the microbiome-gut-brain axis succinctly. "There is a long and winding path ahead of those scientists brave enough to investigate the strange reality of the microbiome-gut-brain axis. No doubt a multitude of molecules are involved in various ways to differing degrees.

"In the far-flung future, perhaps medicines specifically targeting the microbiome will be created for psychiatric conditions; the microbiome may become an early warning system for certain diseases or even a diagnostic tool. For now, all we can do is ponder the influence that bacteria have on our everyday state of mind. We should also be amazed and amused that humans, as intelligent as we consider ourselves, are partially under the control of single-celled lifeforms."

You can see how important it is for women, as Golden Gates, to educate ourselves, each other, our children and our future generations. Our future depends on taking care of the gut bacteria within us and the microbiome we pass on to our babies. Our microbiome and our gut microbiota diversity regulate our mood, our hormones, our immune system and our stress levels, and if they are disrupted they can trigger cancer and chronic disease. In short, the trillions of bacteria in your gut hold the key to your physical, hormonal, mental, immune and emotional wellness. I often ponder if our attraction to a mate is the result of our colony of bugs communicating with each other.

So, next time you have that gut feeling, you'll know it's the bugs in your microbiome talking to you. They may just be telling you something you need to hear.

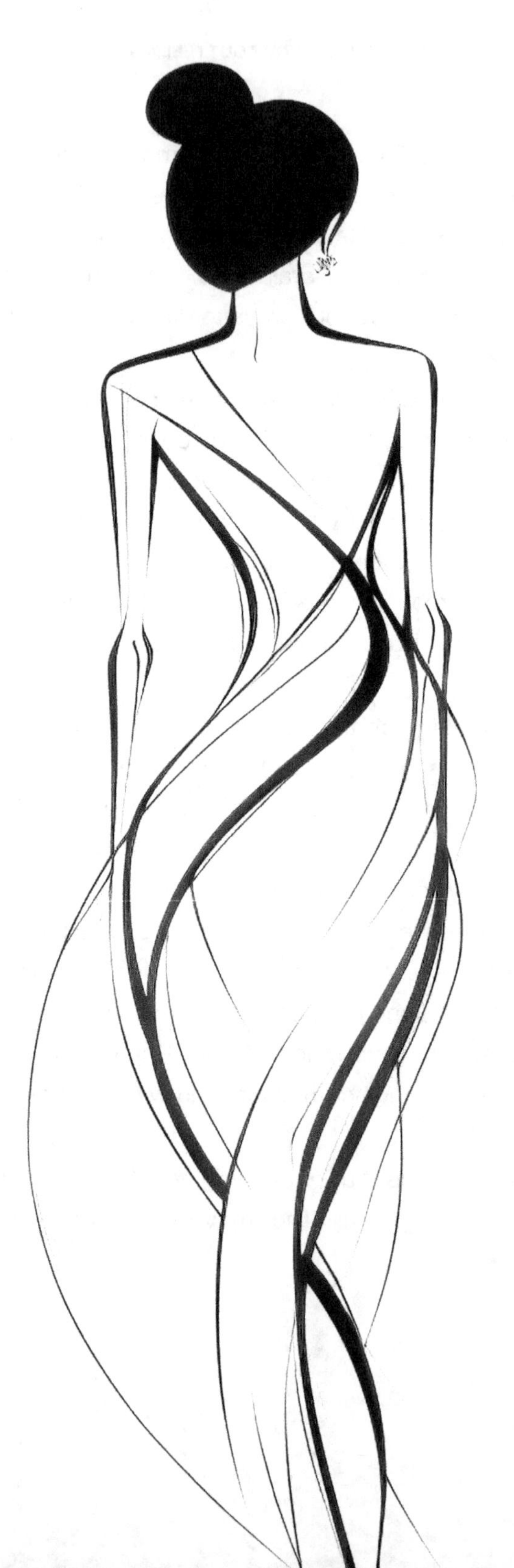

Chapter 12

The Hormone Hierarchy

"If I love you, I need not
continually speak
of my love – you will know
without any words."

'Abdu'l–Bahá, Paris Talks

Our hormones are chemical messengers produced by the different glands in our bodies. They play an intricate and significant role in every aspect of our wellbeing and our relationships, and affect every cell and every system in the body.

Hormones influence how we behave, think, feel, function, remember and react. They affect our mood, our digestion, our capacity for growth and learning, and perhaps even our spirit and soul. The interactions and the intricate balance between our hormones play a vital role in our wellbeing, as well as an important function in longevity. If one hormone has a more dominant relationship to another, it creates inflammation that triggers dysfunction, degeneration, and disease.

The overall system of the hormones produced by our bodies is a complex hierarchy. The highest glands in the body are the hypothalamus and pituitary in the brain. These glands release and produce a number of hormones, but for the purposes of discussing longevity, oxytocin is the player. The hormones produced by the thyroid gland at the front of the neck are next in the line-up. Then the stress hormones produced by the adrenal glands, such as cortisol, and the pancreatic hormone, insulin, compete for third place in the hierarchy. The pancreas sits on the left side of the upper abdomen, under the spleen, while the adrenal glands sit at the back of the body above the kidneys.

Insulin and cortisol perform an extremely powerful dance together. The release of stress hormones can trigger insulin production, and vice-versa. Both these hormones in turn influence the regulation of the next set of hormones: testosterone, progesterone, and estrogens. Usually called the sex hormones, these are produced by the ovaries in women, by the testicles in men.

The higher-level hormones take priority over lower-level hormones – and this hierarchy of hormones is important when it comes to improving your symptoms, reducing health risks and optimizing wellbeing. Think of it like your family tree. Your parents must get together before you are conceived, and you must get together with your partner before your children are conceived. That is the natural order. The same is true with hormones. Oxytocin comes first before thyroid hormones, adrenal hormones, and insulin. And, finally, testosterone, estrogen, and progesterone are produced.

Because of this hierarchy, I find that higher-level hormones must be addressed and balanced first, before lower-level hormones. In other words, if you address only estrogen, a lower-level hormone, during menopause, you may not achieve the hormonal health you are seeking. Think about the hierarchy of the process of a baby developing. Before and just after birth, oxytocin, the cuddle hormone, is needed for proper nurturing of the newborn baby. As the baby grows, the thyroid becomes more active, followed by the pancreas and adrenal glands. It is not until puberty that the sex glands are activated to produce sex hormones.

So, when you want to balance and support hormones during menopause, I find most people feel much healthier when their higher-level hormones, such as oxytocin and the thyroid, adrenal and pancreatic hormones, are supported before the sex hormones. Let's explain these hormones in more depth.

Oxytocin: The Love Hormone

Human interaction is one of our most vital needs for ensuring our survival and wellbeing. Hugging, listening and having close relationships with others activate one of the key hormones required for longevity: oxytocin, also known as the 'love' or 'cuddle' hormone.

Oxytocin is produced by the hypothalamus and released by the pituitary gland when our baby is born, but its impact goes much further than promoting parent-infant bonding. The release of oxytocin triggers the regulation of the autonomic nervous system, the immune system and the release of the relaxation chemicals. Oxytocin can also regulate the hypothalamus-pituitary-axis (HPA), which helps us manage stress more appropriately.

Since oxytocin affects the nervous system and is made up of complex proteins, it belongs to a class of complex proteins called neuropeptides. Oxytocin helps us build bonds of trust. It activates proper stress response during trauma, illness, anxiety and chronic stress. It creates an automatic sense of generosity, forgiveness, security, joy and psychological stability within us. Low oxytocin levels increase the risk for depression, anxiety, schizophrenia, and borderline personality. Furthermore, low oxytocin levels in the mother have been linked to autism in the child[1], who can be effectively treated with oxytocin therapy.

Oxytocin maintains normal blood pressure while inhibiting levels of stress hormones, such as cortisol. Its anti-inflammatory effects help with pain, and it has a powerful bonding effect on human relationships. If you have nursed a child, you may remember the sensation you had just before your milk 'let down'. Your nervous system had to relax to allow the milk to release every time the baby sucked. This was the work of oxytocin.

Breast milk secretion occurs when oxytocin is released in response to nipple stimulation. While oxytocin activates the secretion of breast milk, it also helps suppress breast cancer[2] and ovarian cancer[3], creating more resilience[4]. In fact, the longer a woman nurses, the lower her risk of breast cancer[5] and ovarian cancer[6]. I often prescribe oxytocin to cancer patients and those with chronic diseases to support their immune system, their nervous system, their stress response and, of course, to help suppress the growth of their cancer.

The mother doesn't lose bone density while making breast milk – despite the huge amounts of nutrition and minerals needed – because oxytocin is the key supporter for bone density. It directly impacts bone mineralization, helping increase bone mass to build stronger bones[7].

As we get older, it is important for both women and men to maintain elevated oxytocin levels. Oxytocin has been linked to protecting us against accelerated aging and improves the regeneration of aged tissue stem cells, including muscle cells and heart cells[8,9]. It also suppresses appetite by dampening the brain's food-reward system[10] and therefore plays a role in maintaining healthy body weight, leaner muscle mass and higher bone density.

For those with higher inflammation and chronic pain, oxytocin can act as a natural anti-inflammatory, pain reducer[11] and immune regulator[12]. Melatonin, our sleep hormone, makes us more sensitive to oxytocin[13]. So, when you are in pain, instead of reaching for that Tylenol or Ibuprofen, try getting more sleep, giving someone a hug, or incorporating some of the ways to increase your oxytocin levels that I've listed in the next table.

Oxytocin has a snowball effect: the more oxytocin is activated and available to cells, the more oxytocin is produced and released from the pituitary gland in the brain. Think about the effects of the hug you may give someone. That hug activates the production of oxytocin for both of you for hours, assisting your wellbeing and longevity. Furthermore, oxytocin interacts with and affects the balance of other hormones within the body such as cortisol, dopamine, and estrogen – all of which impact behavior, stress, and physical and emotional wellbeing.

Ways to Increase Oxytocin

- Hugging, touching and cuddling
- Socializing
- Petting a dog, cat or any pet
- Nursing
- Positive self-talk, or complimenting others
- Sexual stimulation/romantic relationships
- Listening or playing soothing music
- Warm showers or acute cold exposure
- Charitable behavior
- Storytelling
- Empathy towards strangers
- Belonging to a community
- Eye-contact, laughing
- Altruistic actions, such as cooking for someone or sharing a meal
- Aromatherapy using essential oils of jasmine, lavender, chamomile, clary sage, Indian sandalwood, or neroli
- Vitamin D, magnesium, vitamin C, taurine
- Fenugreek
- Genistein from organic soy

Oxytocin is released when we feel a sense of belonging. When we create environments that provide positive social interactions, especially through giving unconditionally, we activate oxytocin release in all parties involved. Have you noticed how elated you may feel when you cook a meal for a loved one or a friend, or when you involve yourself in charitable work? This is because your actions of creating community through service stimulate the release of oxytocin.

Each time I come back from a weekend meeting of the Mona Foundation's Board of Directors, for instance, I feel a high. That high, a result of oxytocin and dopamine release, brings me a sense of peace, joy, and emotional security because I am involving myself in volunteer work to educate children.

I remember visiting some of the schools the Mona Foundation supports in India just before the pandemic hit.

The pure act of visiting these schoolkids, seeing the innocent joy and gratitude on the faces of those children, and knowing they were shown kindness, love and support, made my heart sing. Not once did I get sick there. Not once did I feel tired and overwhelmed. Instead, there was a sense of peace, relaxation and elevation. I believe a major reason for this was oxytocin doing its work to create peace and wellbeing within me, my travel companions, and those children.

You may now understand the importance of addressing oxytocin first in the hierarchy, before any other hormone. I recommend that we all intentionally engage in acts of kindness, service and community-building to promote the release of our love hormone to boost our individual and collective wellbeing and youthful aging.

The Thyroid Queen

Next in the hormone line-up is the thyroid, a heart-shaped gland that sits in front of the windpipe. I like to refer to the thyroid as the 'queen' of all glands because it sits highest in the body apart from the pituitary and hypothalamus found in the brain. The queen regulates almost everything in the body: from signaling to the adrenal glands and ovaries to release their hormones to regulating our metabolism, cell function, body temperature, immune system and digestion.

The thyroid has a hand in almost everything that goes on in the body. It interacts closely with stress hormones like cortisol and insulin, the pancreatic hormone. The thyroid can be affected by our thoughts, diet, lifestyle, emotions and sex hormones. When the thyroid slows down our energy drops, monthly cycles become irregular, depression sets in, sleep gets disturbed, brain function slows, eyebrows thin on the ends, skin dries and constipation ensues. The thyroid sits in the throat chakra and can be responsible for our ability to speak our truth. When we suppress our voice, our truth, we energetically suppress the thyroid gland from functioning properly.

The thyroid requires multiple nutrients to function properly: chiefly vitamin B6, iodine, selenium, zinc, copper, iron and tyrosine. Being deficient in any of these nutrients can weaken thyroid hormone function leading to hypothyroidism (low thyroid). Because the thyroid and adrenal glands (the stress regulator glands) have a close relationship, when one is stressed, the other overcompensates. Therefore, both need to be supported when one shows up on tests and the other doesn't.

When the immune system is fighting viruses or parasites, becomes toxic with metals[14], or is stressed by food intolerances such as dairy and gluten[15], the immune system can become 'allergic' to the thyroid gland

and begins attacking it. We call this condition Hashimoto's thyroiditis, or autoimmune thyroiditis. Hashimoto's may also be triggered during perimenopause, when estrogen and progesterone levels begin to drop, and estrogen starts to dominate over progesterone[16]. The presence of Hashimoto's can be the initial warning sign of an increased risk for breast cancer.

Since the COVID-19 pandemic, I have seen a significantly higher incidence of patients with Hashimoto's thyroiditis because the COVID-19 virus, or its vaccine, induce a general autoimmune dysregulation, placing stress on the thyroid-adrenal relationship[17]. Dormant chronic infections, like the Epstein-Barr virus, may also reactivate as a result.

Signs and Symptoms of Hypothyroidism

- Brain fog and memory issues
- Constipation or irritable bowel syndrome
- Depression or lack of motivation
- Delayed Achilles tendon reflex
- Dizziness/near-fainting spells
- Dry skin and brittle hair
- Elevated cholesterol
- Fatigue
- Fatty liver
- Fertility issues
- Generalized hair thinning and hair loss
- Generalized weight gain or difficulty losing weight
- Goiter
- Hypoglycemia
- Irregular or heavy menstruation
- Muscle aches and/or heaviness
- Puffy face and/or puffy lower eyelids
- Thinning eyebrows at the ends

In medicine, doctors are trained to test thyroid mainly by ordering TSH (thyroid stimulating hormone) and Free T4 (free inactive thyroid hormone). Because the majority of the active thyroid hormone, free T3, is produced mainly in the tissues from converting T4 to T3 and not in the thyroid gland itself, testing for only TSH and Free T4 is usually insufficient to identify thyroid dysfunction. Most thyroid conditions get missed as a result.

Hence, I often order TSH, FT4, FT3, Reverse T3 and Thyroid antibodies along with a DUTCH hormone urine and saliva test to look at all the female, male and adrenal hormones, their metabolites, and some key nutrients. This more comprehensive approach helps identify a more complete picture of the thyroid function, hidden thyroid imbalances and other related hormone conditions.

When it comes to healing the thyroid queen, modern synthetic thyroid medications are often not enough. This is because they further suppress thyroid function and emotions, forcing the pathophysiology of the illness even deeper, especially in premenopausal women[18]. In postmenopausal women, over-treatment or hyperthyroidism can result in increased risk of breast cancer[19].

I believe that to properly heal the thyroid, the underlying root causes must be addressed. For example, we must identify hidden infections, toxic metals and suppressed and blocked emotions and thoughts. Profound emotions hidden within the thyroid often convey the lineage of controlled silence passed on to women through their maternal bloodline. These repressed feelings can be acknowledged and released through therapy, relieving the stress held in the throat and thyroid.

Alongside emotional release work, we must also perform a nutrient, diet and lifestyle evaluation. Supplementing iodine, tyrosine, selenium, vitamin B6, and zinc – the nutrients involved in producing thyroid hormones – can help to restore thyroid function[20]. If a temporary prescription medication is required until the underlying causes have been addressed, I prefer to prescribe desiccated thyroid, a natural thyroid containing both T4 and T3, as well as T2, and T1 thyroid hormones, from either a bovine or porcine source. Contrary to common belief, I have found most patients are able to wean off desiccated thyroid medication as the thyroid heals. Weaning off synthetic thyroid hormones, such as Levothyroxine or Synthroid, is much more difficult but not impossible under proper medical guidance.

Making small dietary modifications can make a big difference to thyroid function. For instance, excessive amounts of *raw* cruciferous vegetables, such as broccoli, cauliflower and cabbage, contain thiocyanates. These chemicals compete with thyroid hormone function and iodine uptake and slow thyroid function down. Slightly steaming or cooking the vegetables destroys thiocyanates, reducing the stress on the thyroid while supporting healthy estrogen metabolism. Soy products, especially soymilk and tofu, contain soy isoflavones which appear to slow thyroid function transiently for up to 3 months and then return to normal by six months[21].

Seaweed and kelp are fantastic for thyroid function because they contain naturally occurring iodine. However, do make sure to purchase low mercury, organic seaweed. Iodized table salt contains sodium chloride sprayed with iodate, and overconsumption can cause an array of thyroid toxicity symptoms[22]. Naturally occurring iodine can be found in Himalayan salt and trace mineral sea salt. For a list of therapeutic treatments to treat thyroid conditions, and a list of foods to help support thyroid function, please refer to GoldenGateBook.com/resources.

Insulin: The Sugar Regulator

The silent epidemic of our modern-day society is insulin resistance, also known as metabolic syndrome or prediabetes. The epidemic of obesity among adults and children, usually a by-product of insulin resistance, springs from our toxic food and lifestyle practices.

Modern inventions have made our bodies toxic, reactive and insulin-resistant. They are everywhere we look: processed foods, pesticides and herbicides and chemicals in our food and air, refined sugar, artificial sweeteners, and chemically farmed fish, processed poultry and meats[23]. These toxins are magnified by the stress created by our environment: our quick-fix mindset, our materialistic and competitive technology-driven society, and the overload of medications urinated into our drinking water systems, among many other modern-day stressors.

These 21st century villains create stress within the body and often harbor in glands like the pancreas, where insulin forms. Stress hormones, such as cortisol, that are released by our adrenal glands in response to these toxic stressors activate the release of sugar from our sugar stores. A rise in blood sugar, which is inflammatory, activates the release of insulin, which is anti-inflammatory, in an attempt to reduce inflammaging and blood sugar levels. When blood sugar drops as a result of high insulin, cortisol responds to this stress, leading to more sugar being released. This vicious cycle leads to insulin resistance causing inflammation, weight gain, fatigue, brain fog and sleep disturbances[24]. It increases the risks of chronic pain[25], depression[26], anxiety, hormonal imbalances, autoimmune disease[27], chronic infections, diabetes, mitochondrial dysfunction[28], heart disease, dementia[29] and cancer[30].

Imagine ten people lined up at the bus stop. The people in this analogy represent sugar. They call for a bus (insulin) from the bus depot (the pancreas) to take them to their workplace (the cells). The bus comes by, but only picks up one person. The nine remaining people call for another bus. Meanwhile, more people join the line-up at the bus stop. Another bus comes, but it only picks up three people. After a while, lots of people (sugars) wait at the bus stop while the buses (insulin) resist picking them up and block the roadway (the arteries). This is known as insulin resistance and leads to heart disease, stroke, diabetes and cancer. Eventually, the bus depot runs out of buses and the road (the blood) fills up with people (sugars). This is called diabetes.

Insulin resistance is often difficult to identify and even those of us who may seem to have relatively healthy diets and weight may be diagnosed with insulin resistance. Insulin resistance is the most common modern-day condition among all age-groups causing inflammation. Many of my patients are often shocked to find out that they have insulin resistance, even though they do not eat sugar, eat relatively healthy diets and/or are not overweight.

Insulin resistance, like I mentioned earlier, doesn't just come from sugar and bad food. Lifestyle practices including nutrient toxicity (overeating) and the biggest toxin of them all, stress, are its silent feeders[31,32]. We all know stress comes from our chosen reactions and mental outlook in life, but stress can also be created within our bodies. For example, skipping meals, eating too late, fasting too long, not getting enough sleep, drinking alcohol, starting the morning with carbohydrates, being exposed to chemicals and electromagnetic radiation fields, and harboring emotional baggage potentially promote insulin resistance over time[33].

We have the capacity to correct insulin sensitivity through being aware of our stressors and addressing those that trigger our internal fight-and-flight response. We can incorporate mindful practices regarding our food, lifestyle practices and toxic exposures to reduce our bodies' risk of inflammation, diabetes, heart disease and cancer.

You can find some therapeutic practices you may wish to incorporate into your lifestyle to optimize insulin sensitivity and regulate blood sugar and insulin levels on **GoldenGateBook.com/resources**. For instance, therapeutic fasting, which we will discuss in Virtue III, can be a powerful tool to reset insulin resistance and blood sugar. For some of my patients, I prescribe a continuous glucose monitor (CGM), which they wear on their belly or the back of their upper arm to monitor blood sugar levels. By using a CGM, they learn what foods, eating habits, meal schedules, exercise regimes, and sleeping habits work best for them to regulate their blood sugar, which in turn supports healthier insulin function.

Stress, Sex, Sugar and Salt

Your adrenal glands, the triangular glands sitting above the kidneys, normally release the four "S" hormones: stress, sugar, sex and salt-balancing hormones. The role of the adrenal glands is to secrete these hormones as needed to balance your blood sugar, stress reactions, sexual energies, blood pressure and fluid accumulation. During menopause, the adrenal glands take over the role of ovaries in producing sex hormones.

Adrenal hormones, like cortisol, are what kick in when you wake up so you get out of bed standing upright without falling over. When cortisol is not kicking in because you are burnt out, you may experience episodes of dizziness, lightheadedness and near-fainting spells. During perimenopause, the regulation and release of these hormones from the adrenal glands becomes chaotic, especially if you are not mindful of your lifestyle, dietary, and spiritual habits. Burnt out adrenal glands may not be able to support the extra role of taking on the production of sex hormones during perimenopause. Hence, the challenge of the transition may make you may feel tired, fat, dizzy, stressed and no longer sexy.

Stress hormones, like cortisol and DHEA, act to reduce inflammation in the body. When cortisol is high during prenatal maternal stress, or when the environment around a baby is stressful, inducing high cortisol in the infant, the baby's genetics, brain function and behavior, methylation function and the microbiome shift, promoting more inflammatory and allergic conditions, and other adverse conditions and behaviors in the newborn[34]. The stress intolerance and cellular changes in the newborn may lead to a lifetime's challenge of stress-related immune conditions, like eczema, asthma, allergies and autoimmune disease[35]. When the baby girl grows up and enters menopause with the lower reserves of stress hormones, the changes in methylation and vitamin D receptors make menopause challenging.

These alterations in gene expression as a result of environmental influences is called epigenetics. We now know that such epigenetic alterations are passed on to grandchildren, increasing certain health risks in the future generations. These grandchildren have higher risks of heart disease, for example, as a result of the alterations in vitamin B12, D receptors and methylation in response to stressors, such as immigration and racism experienced by grandma[36]. This is called transgenerational epigenetic inheritance. However, the good news is that supplementation with curcumin, sulforaphane and butyrate[37], as well as meditation[38], fasting and regular exercise[39], can potentially modify and correct some of these epigenetic alterations, to reduce health risks for ourselves and future generations.

Melatonin: The Sleeping Beauty Hormone

Sleep is the most important bodily activity required for health, wellbeing, and slowing aging. Those who get the best sleep usually have optimum levels of melatonin, a neurohormone released by the pineal gland. Melatonin is made from the amino acid tryptophan, which maintains the circadian rhythm and is vital for maintaining overall health.

Melatonin is synthesized, taken up, utilized and present in high concentrations in the mitochondria, the powerhouse of cells. It protects the mitochondria from oxidative stress and damage, from aging[40]. Melatonin is therefore one of the most powerful antiaging tools known to humanity. As senescence cells (cells growing old that indicate aging) set in with age, melatonin therapy can potentially reverse the detrimental effects of senescence cells[41].

Every organ in the body has melatonin receptors (MT1 and MT2). These include the brain, the heart and arteries, the digestive tract, the liver, gallbladder, breasts, prostate, ovaries, placenta, kidneys, and white and brown fat cells. In other words, melatonin impacts almost every major cell and organ in the body. Low levels of this important neurohormone are associated with the worst health outcomes and several modern-day diseases, as was shown in a small study of 37 critically ill patients[42]. Sufficient melatonin levels protect cells against toxicity, infections, cellular damage and aging. But melatonin's magical powers don't stop there. In summary:

- Melatonin supports mitochondria health supporting healthier aging and beautiful skin and hair[43].

- Melatonin acts as an immune modulator, an anti-inflammatory and an antioxidant protecting heart cells from free radical damage[44]. It appears to offer protection against heart disease, hypertension, and high cholesterol[45].

- Melatonin is involved in our immune response to infections, including parasitic infections. Melatonin therapy may also be used to treat recurrent genital herpes[46].

- Melatonin closely interacts with ghrelin, leptin, and insulin to reduce obesity, diabetes and metabolic syndrome[47]. Night-shift nurses have an increased risk of metabolic syndrome and chronic diseases because of lower melatonin levels[48].

- Melatonin therapy is a powerful treatment for sarcopenia[49].

- When melatonin is low, there is more inflammation and oxidative stress damage in the heart and blood sugar and insulin levels tend to increase, leading to increased risk of neurodegenerative conditions like dementia, Alzheimer's[50] and Parkinson's[51].

- Melatonin therapy helps the body's anti-inflammatory and anti-oxidant systems protect the nervous system from degenerating[52].

- Because of its neuroprotective qualities, melatonin therapy can treat patients with concussion and traumatic brain injuries[53].

- High levels of melatonin appear to inhibit the initiation, progression, and metastasis of cancer. To support cancer patients, I often prescribe at least 40 mg of melatonin per day and counsel them on getting good sleep[54].

- For easy ways to increase melatonin, see my website GoldenGateBook.com/resources.

As you can see, making sure our body's complex system of hormones is balanced plays a major role in our wellbeing. Without balanced hormones, we may often lack the determination, motivation and energy to be the Golden Gates we are meant to be. We age more quickly. We become stiffer. Our minds weaken. Our capacity to function in this world slows. And we get sicker.

The more balanced your hormones, on the other hand, the better you cultivate your health and the more productively you function. And one of the most potent tools for aging gracefully and youthfully is improving your melatonin levels and making sure you get enough sleep. Now you know the science behind the expression "get your beauty sleep".

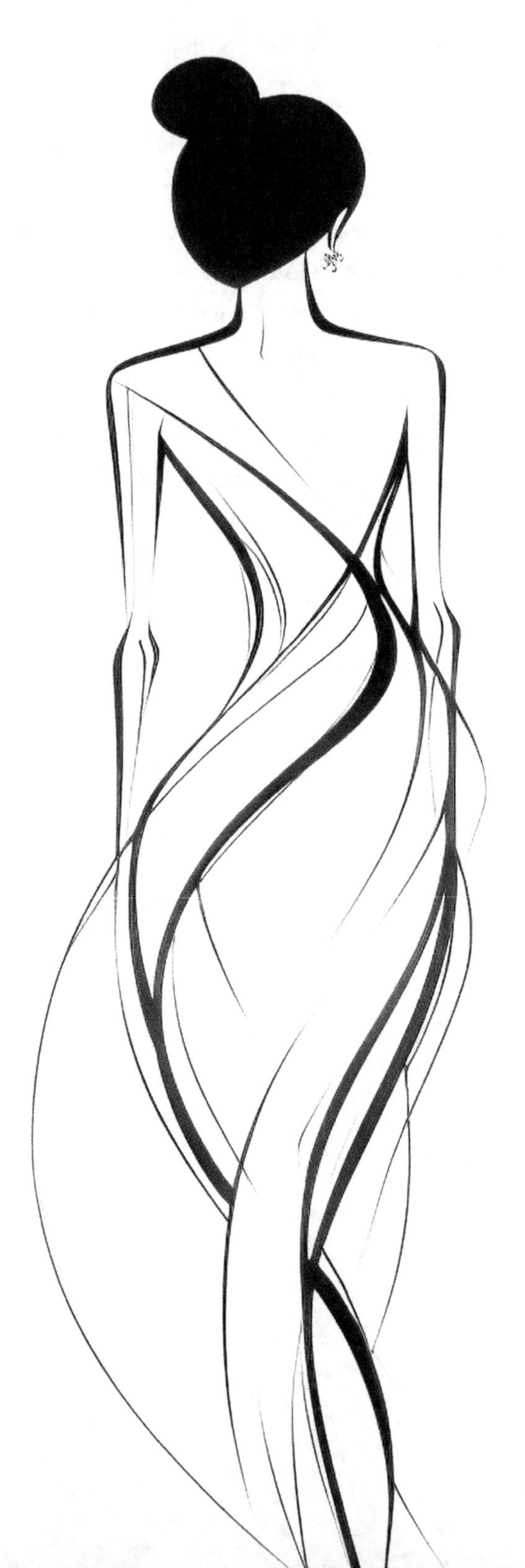

Chapter 13

The
Sex
Hormones

"Where there is love,
nothing is too much
trouble, and there
is always time."

'Abdu'l-Bahá

Women have more than 50 different hormones – and their ebbs and flows and their interactions are far more complex than the male hormonal system.

Each month we experience a rollercoaster ride as our hormones oscillate through each monthly cycle: elevated estrogen levels in the first half of the cycle, coupled with higher levels of progesterone in the second half. While these monthly cycles can be challenging enough, we then have to contend with the immense hormonal shifts during perimenopause and menopause – a time of crisis and victories as our mind and body we once knew morph into new ways of being.

Progesterone, produced by the corpus luteum in the ovaries, is the dominant hormone in the second half of our cycle. During our fertile years, progesterone prepares the body for pregnancy by promoting the growth of the uterine lining. Progesterone levels remain high during pregnancy to help maintain the uterine lining and pregnancy while preventing labor contractions. Progesterone is also involved in the development of the fetus, helping to regulate the growth and function of the placenta.

In our modern-day, high-stress society, progesterone deficiency is one of the main causes of infertility and spontaneous miscarriages because progesterone is also involved with stress management. Low levels can contribute to menstrual irregularities, infertility and an increased risk of miscarriage[1]. High or low levels of progesterone can cause symptoms such as bloating, mood changes and fatigue, especially during the second half of a woman's cycle.

In addition to its reproductive functions, progesterone plays an essential role in regulating mood, promoting healthy sleep, maintaining strong bone density and keeping our cardiovascular system healthy.

It has neuroprotective qualities, meaning it protects the nervous system from inflammation and degeneration, and it is involved in regulating our immune system.

Progesterone is also a calming hormone. It activates the parasympathetic nervous system to reduce anxiety and support sleep, digestion and more. Many people who experienced COVID-19 symptoms or related vaccinations in conjunction with higher stress levels during the pandemic may have lower amounts of progesterone relative to estrogen, known as estrogen dominance[2], or disturbed hormonal balance[3]. This has become a major contributing factor to the higher amounts of anxiety, insomnia, and mental health issues many have experienced during and since the pandemic.

Progesterone, the natural hormone produced by the body, is often confused with progestin, a chemically synthesized pharmaceutical hormone. When I speak about progesterone in this book, I am referring to the hormone naturally produced by the body or the bio-identical hormone, which comes from plants such as wild yams. Natural progesterone, and not progestin, has been associated with lower risks of cancer[4] and high blood pressure[5], improved bone health[6] and reduction in anxiety[7,8]. Progestin, the pharmaceutically synthesized compound, on the other hand, often acts in the opposite way: progestins potentially increase cancer risks and inflammation, leading to increased risk of heart disease, especially when combined with synthetic estrogen[9].

During perimenopause and menopause, progesterone production is the first to slow as the ovaries begin to stop functioning. In periods of high stress during perimenopause or menopause, progesterone may also be redeployed to produce cortisol, the main fight-and-flight hormone. This is called progesterone steal. Put simply, progesterone is stolen from its reproductive function to meet the demands of stress management by supporting cortisol production.

Reduced production and increased demand for progesterone during perimenopause and menopause means progesterone levels drop significantly. As a result, women often experience sleep disturbances, increased anxiety, restless leg syndrome, early-stage bone loss, stress intolerance and so much more. Supporting progesterone levels during perimenopause and periods of high stress often improves sleep quality, reduces anxiety, and even increases bone re-mineralization.

Ways to support progesterone include consuming foods that act as phytoprogestins (act as progesterones), such as apigenin from chamomile, naringenin in citrus fruit, luteolin found in over 300 plants[10], wild yams, and evening primrose oil[11], sunflower seeds, chickpeas[12] and sesame seeds. Practicing meditation, yoga, deep-breathing exercises and engaging in mild to moderate exercise support progesterone levels too, because they help reduce stress and, therefore, minimizing progesterone steal.

Testosterone: not just for men

Testosterone is often seen as a male hormone, but it plays a major role in a female's body. In fact, second to thyroid hormones, testosterone is the most abundant active hormone in the body during the lifespan of a woman. Yes, we have more testosterone than estrogen or progesterone, ladies. Testosterone receptors are found in nearly every tissue of our bodies: in the breasts, uterus, brain, heart, nervous system, blood vessels, digestive tract, bladder, ovaries, endocrine glands, vaginal tissue, skin, bone, bone marrow, muscle and adipose tissue. Testosterone is necessary not only for general wellbeing but also for decision-making, libido, mood, and muscle and bone mass[13].

In most women, as testosterone levels gradually drop with aging, testosterone therapy can be an effective and safe treatment for menopausal symptoms – especially as pellets[14,15] of bio-identical testosterone placed under the skin, or as a topical hormone cream applied vaginally[16]. The rate of early mortality is higher in women who are deficient in testosterone or vitamin D, a neuro-endocrine hormone[17]. Initial data on pellet therapy shows it has a promising effect on reducing the rate of breast cancer and protecting women against early mortality[18]. However, testosterone therapy for women has not yet been approved by the Food and Drug Administration.

Estrogen: The Good, the Bad and the Ugly

The hormone ride gets a little more complex when we consider estrogens, a group of pretty important hormones that are responsible for the development and regulation of female reproduction organs and other significant biological processes in the body.

Estrogen plays a crucial role in the development of female secondary sexual characteristics, such as breast development and the growth of pubic hair. It also regulates the menstrual cycle, thickens the uterine lining in preparation for pregnancy, and regulates metabolism and inflammation. Emerging data illustrates the importance of estrogens in men as well: it has a hand in male fertility, sperm production and sexual function, as well as regulating insulin and blood sugar balance and possible other physiological functions[19].

Outside the reproductive system, estrogens support healthy bones by preventing bone loss, they regulate cholesterol levels, and they affect our mood, our cognitive function, and the health of our skin, brain and heart[20]. Most importantly they activate the antioxidant system in our mitochondria, our cell's main energy engine[21], and they modulate heart physiology and protect the brain against aging[22]. Estrogens also activate gene expression and cellular communication[23]. This explains why our cells' engines weaken when estrogen levels decline during perimenopause.

The human body produces three types of estrogen, which I have labeled the good, the bad and the ugly. The ugly estrogen is called estrone (E1), which is the most genotoxic estrogen, meaning toxic to our genes, because it has the strongest association with cancer and inflammation[24]. Estriol (E3) is the good estrogen because it is the weakest and safest estrogen[25]. The bad estrogen is estradiol (E2), which is the most dominant form of estrogen in our bodies and is mostly produced by the ovaries, with secondary supply from the adrenal glands.

In reality, estradiol has a positive effect most of the time, but I have called it the bad estrogen because E2 can turn ugly depending on your genetics and your epigenetics – that is, your lifestyle practices and environmental exposures – impacting its metabolism. Here is a more detailed fact-file on the three types of estrogen:

Estrone (E1)

Estrone (E1) is a weak but the most genotoxic of all estrogens. It is mainly produced when androgens (male hormones) are converted to E1 in body fat after menopause. E1 is associated with higher risks of breast cancers and other hormone-related cancers in post-menopausal women, because it stimulates inflammation and can break down into 4-OH-E1, an even more dangerous estrogen by-product that damages DNA[26].

When 4-OH-E1 is properly methylated to 4-MeE1, it is easily eliminated and cancer risks are reduced. However, when it is not methylated properly and instead builds up, it turns into 3,4-quinones, chemicals which are carcinogenic[27]. Supporting glutathione can reduce DNA damage caused by 4-OH-E1.

Body composition makes a difference when it comes to cancer risks. Those with high body fat and lower muscle mass (called sarcopenia) have increased risk of cancer and mortality[28]. Increased body fat around the waist, arms and legs in postmenopausal women is associated with higher risk of cancer[29], perhaps because of E1 conversion.

Higher body fat increases other inflammatory hormones as well, such as adiponectin, IL-6, and c-reactive protein, which further add insult to inflammation, insulin-resistance and higher risks of hormone-related cancers[30]. Improving muscle mass and reducing body fat, especially after menopause, helps reduce cancer risks – perhaps because it reduces estrogen-related toxins that can potentially build up in body fat.

Estradiol (E2)

Estradiol (E2) is the most potent and prevalent estrogen in the body, commonly found as 17 beta-estradiol. Estradiol is most active during the first half of a woman's menstrual cycle, and it mainly impacts the health of our bones, heart, skin, and brain. It protects the heart and blood vessels, it plays a part in maintaining the body's anti-inflammatory and antioxidant systems, and it can potentially change gene expression[31].

As 17 beta-estradiol, it supports healthy cholesterol levels and cognitive function and reduces plaque build-up in arteries[32]. Estradiol is also regarded as an anabolic hormone because it builds muscle and tissue, including the lining of the uterus, and helps to lubricate joints and ensure tendons and ligaments stay flexible[33]. This is why we may wake up in the morning feeling achy and stiff as estradiol levels decline in perimenopause and menopause.

Estriol (E3)

Estriol (E3) is produced in very small amounts, primarily by the placenta, as well as by the fetal liver and our adrenal glands. It does not convert to 4-OH-E1 and is associated with cancer-protective qualities. Estrogen-related cancer risks are lower during pregnancy partly perhaps because there is more protective estriol roaming in the body, peaking in the third trimester. During pregnancy, estriol helps promote the development of the placenta and the fetus.

Several years ago, I diagnosed Tonya, a 38-year-old woman who was two months pregnant, with an aggressive triple-negative breast cancer. Her oncologist told her she needed to start chemo as soon as possible, otherwise both she and her baby would not survive the pregnancy. Tonya ignored her oncologist's recommendation and instead pursued supportive cancer care with me, practicing healthy nutrition, lifestyle, meditation and supplementation. Contrary to her oncologist's belief, her cancer did not grow or spread during her pregnancy. Instead, she thrived and delivered her baby perfectly on time as nature intended.

My hypothesis for her survival during pregnancy was partially due to the higher levels of estriol during her pregnancy.

Estriol therapy may also be used to treat menopausal symptoms and conditions such as osteoporosis[34] or multiple sclerosis[35]. In these cases, it is typically used in combination with other hormones, such as estradiol and progesterone. Because estriol is much weaker than other estrogens, it has a lower risk[36] of causing some of the side effects historically associated with synthetic estrogen therapy, especially when pulsed[37].

We now recognize that estrogens also play a dominant role in the development, function and protection of the brain and central nervous system. Because of this important role, when estrogen levels drop during perimenopause, memory and cognitive function become significantly impaired. This is why we sometimes feel brain-fogged, or experience forgetfulness, at times during perimenopause and menopause[38]. Women experiencing early menopause before the age of 45, or those who experience surgically induced menopause, tend to have a higher risk of dementia while those experiencing menopause after 55 have a significantly lower risk of dementia[39].

When we put all this together, the picture shows that when estrogen levels, particularly estradiol, drop during perimenopause, we experience more fatigue, memory issues, and joint pain and stiffness, plus higher cholesterol and inflammation, increased belly fat, decreased bone density and saggy skin. In other words, we feel old, stiff, depressed, tired, forgetful and fat.

To make matters worse, all these symptoms can literally occur overnight, because estradiol levels can drop quickly during the last months of perimenopause. When we feel hot flushes, or see wrinkles on our skin, we are experiencing the oxidative stress resulting from lower levels of estrogen. Getting Botox or a facelift to cover up our wrinkles will not fix the root of the problem: the inflammation caused by the drop in estradiol levels.

To truly slow the aging process in our cells, our brains, and our cardiovascular symptom, we must address the underlying estrogen deficiency. We can do this either through bio-identical estrogen hormone therapy or by increasing our intake of foods that act like estrogen, known as phytoestrogens. Studies suggest phytoestrogen, such as genistein from soy, improve mitochondria function, especially in the heart, while increasing glutathione content in the mitochondria[40]. Genistein, an isoflavone found in high amounts in soybean, chickpeas and fava beans, has been shown to help brain development and function, improve bone healing and mimic estrogens[41].

Genistein has antioxidant, anticancer, anti-inflammatory, antibacterial, antiviral and antidiabetic properties. It acts to reduce inflammation, cancer metastasis, and oxidative stress, among other protective mechanisms[42]. In other words, genistein helps fight inflammation, protect our mitochondria and support the longevity of our cells. So, don't be afraid of soy but do make sure to consume organic soy, and preferably sprouted soy. Try combining it with mushrooms to reduce further your breast cancer risks[43]. One of my favorite foods to start my morning while supporting healthy estrogen, cholesterol and blood sugar/insulin levels and reducing risks of breast cancer is gluten-free miso soup with mushrooms, organic sprouted tofu and organic seaweed. Yum!

Too Much Estrogen Ain't Good!

Women love their estrogens when they are in balance. Healthy estrogen levels make us feel sexy, beautiful and happy. However, when they are out of balance, they can make us sick. Healthy balance of estrogens, and their proper elimination through the liver and the gut, play a vital role in our health, aging and wellbeing.

The ratio of estrogen to progesterone is vital to our health. Sometimes, it is not progesterone that is deficient but estrogen or the unhealthy estrogen metabolites that are elevated. This is known as estrogen dominance[44]: a common modern-day imbalance that increases risks of inflammatory conditions, heart disease and hormone-related cancers such as colon, ovarian, uterine, breast, brain and lung cancers.

Symptoms of Estrogen Dominance

- Brain fog and memory issues in the second half of the cycle
- Endometriosis
- Heavy bleeding or premenstrual spotting
- Irregular cycles
- Mid-cycle and premenstrual fatigue
- Polycystic ovary syndrome (PCOS)
- Premenstrual acne
- Premenstrual bloating, swelling and breast tenderness
- Premenstrual mood swings
- Uterine fibroids and polyps
- Weight gain

Most women with moderate to intense perimenopausal or menopausal symptoms have estrogen dominance, and are at risk for hormone-related inflammatory health conditions and cancer. Insulin resistance often co-occurs with estrogen dominance, as does PCOS (polycystic ovarian syndrome)[45]. We can reduce toxic estrogen metabolites through lifestyle practices of daily sweating in an infrared sauna and daily moderate exercise. Eating foods containing high amounts of sulforaphanes, plus liver-support foods like lemons, artichoke, beets and dandelion root[46], also plays a key role in balancing and metabolizing estrogen, as does regulating our blood sugar, insulin and testosterone levels.

The first stage of estrogen elimination takes place through the liver, incorporating phase I and phase II detoxification. Remember, phase I is like the emptying the fridge of all the old leftovers. Phase II of estrogen elimination is when we pack up the leftovers into garbage bags, and phase III gets the garbage bags out of the house. Phase III takes place in the digestive tract, involving the microbiome, as the garbage is excreted through the colon and the urine.

The process starts when estrogen that has been used by the body travels to the liver through the blood. The liver then breaks down the three forms of estrogen into three metabolites: 2-hydroxyestrone (2-OH-E1), 4-hydroxyesterone (4-OH-E1) and 16-alpha-hydroxyestrone (16-OH-E1). This process is similar to bagging the estrogens into three different garbage bags. The bag containing 2-OH-E1 is the one we want to fill the most because it seems to be the safest and it is thought to protect against inflammation and cancer[47].

The bags containing 4-OH-E1 and 16-OH-E1 are not such healthy bags. In fact, 16-OH-E1 increases cellular proliferation, like in endometriosis, fibroids, breast cysts and benign tumors, while 4-OH-

E1 can lead to DNA damage causing cancer[48]. If our digestive tract does not empty these last two bags properly through phase III, the toxic estrogens re-circulate back into the blood through the colon wall and create more toxicity and more damage in our cells, leading to cancer years later.

So, in a nutshell, you want to make sure your liver makes more 2-hydroxyestrone (2-OH-E1), compared to the other two metabolites. When your liver produces more 2-OH-E1 relative to 4-OH-E1 or 16-OH-E1, the healthier your body and the lower the risks for hormone-related conditions, such as cancer and autoimmune diseases.

For example, higher breast cancer risks are associated with increased ratio of 16-OH-E1 to 2-OH-E1, or higher amounts of 4-OH-E1, which is considered a carcinogen. Foods that support the liver's production of 2-OH-E1 and the elimination of 4-OH-E1 include sulforaphanes from the brassica family, such as cabbage, broccoli sprouts and cauliflower. Quercetin, Indole-3-carbinol and DIM (diindolylmethane) are needed for healthier estrogen metabolism. A healthy gut microbiome is also important for healthy estrogens and their detoxification. You can find a full list of foods to support estrogen metabolism on my website for this book, **GoldenGateBook.com/resources**.

Estradiol and Glutathione

Estradiol protects our cells' mitochondria from being damaged. When estradiol drops during perimenopause, this leads to reduced cellular energy production, decreased glucose metabolism, and damage to the fatty myelin sheaths that protect our nerves[49]. Lower levels of estradiol are accompanied by reduced production of glutathione (GSH), a substance produced by the liver[50]. Glutathione is known as the 'master antioxidant' because it supports the detoxification and elimination of toxic chemicals and carcinogens like 4-OH-E1[51]. During perimenopause, glutathione production drops significantly in women – especially in the mitochondria, the engines of our cells[52]. When glutathione diminishes, the cells and the mitochondria are less protected against oxidative stress, particularly in the heart, liver, and nervous system. Low glutathione causes symptoms like hot flashes and insomnia[53].

We know that the mitochondria inside the lining of the arteries breaks down in direct correlation to estrogen levels dropping during menopause. A decline in estrogen increases the risk for a stroke or a heart attack. The risks can be reduced by starting estrogen therapy as soon as necessary during menopause. Studies also show a direct association between lower estrogen levels and higher risks of dementia and Alzheimer's[54].

The decrease in glutathione production is one of the reasons why menopausal women have a lower detox capacity, heightened sensitivities to foods, chemicals and other toxins, and an increased risk for hormone-related cancers. During perimenopause, my food sensitivities heightened as my estradiol levels declined. I would break out in hives when I ate tomatoes, potatoes, shellfish and rice. But as I became more aware of my body's need to support glutathione production while also supporting estrogen levels, my reactions diminished.

Glutathione is involved not only in detoxification but also in DNA repair, regeneration of vitamins E and C, supporting immune function, neutralizing free radicals, transporting mercury out of the brain and much more[55]. We can boost our glutathione levels by eating foods like avocado, okra, turmeric, asparagus and broccoli containing the amino acids glutamate, glycine and cysteine, which the liver uses to make glutathione[56]. Supplements like N-acetyl-cysteine (NAC), glutamine, omega 3 oils as in flaxseeds or fish oil, vitamins C, E and B2, selenium, and alpha lipoic acid act as co-factors to increase glutathione levels[57]. We can also use intravenous glutathione injections, or glutathione inhalations through a nebulizer[58] or an intranasal spray.

Let's remind ourselves that to fulfil our capacities as Golden Gates, we must not only have strong bodies, but strong minds and joyful spirits too. Therapies that support our hormones, their metabolism and proper detoxification – ranging from modifying our diets and supplementation to bio-identical hormone therapy – provide the building blocks to improving our wellbeing so we can age gracefully and stay healthy for longer. When our hormones are balanced, we can more readily access our inner joy.

Why Am I in Pain?

This pain:
Is it calling me to see that which I don't want to see
Or alerting me to let go of pain that does not belong to me?
My belly hurts, I'm bloated, tired and lonely too
My back heavy, achey so constantly living due
Like I'm pregnant, labored, waiting the unknown
But I'm not, just burdened with a gnawing suit.

I feel the pain, the fear, the worry and the grief
Of my loved one whose pain I wish to take away
But the pain is not mine so what right do I have
To think I'm justified to carry his pain
Thinking I can carry it better than he
While unjustly his right I'm taking with me.

Finding the courage to let go of my own beliefs
Nodding my head quietly in humility
To honor him through journey much needed to grow
I stand perfectly grounded, my two feet rooted for
Holding him as he processes his agony to transform
Consciously learning not to take on his suffering
'Cause it's not mine, not mine to be healing.

As difficult as it may be, I let go to return his pain
Telling him I am here, right here, holding, loving him
I'm committed to accompany him.
He feels safe, supported, ready to release
His long-standing pain
A pain that perhaps does not belong to him.

He finally let's go, throwing away his pain
And now he feels free, me too I am so relieved
Of carrying chronic pain now rightly extinct
With no further no purpose
So empty, so deceased of a home in me.

Surprised I feel and so does he
What happened to the pain, the agony, the weight
Bloating retired, and the back pain departed
'Cause I, we, learnt our lesson to release
A deeper pain that began before our birth
But now serving us simply no longer.

Feeling free, enlightened, joyful, youthful.
Much higher we then begin to resonate
Stronger grows, resilient we become
Our spiritual connection, our beautiful love
Elevating beyond the earthly bond
Intertwined as souls soaring higher towards the Sun.

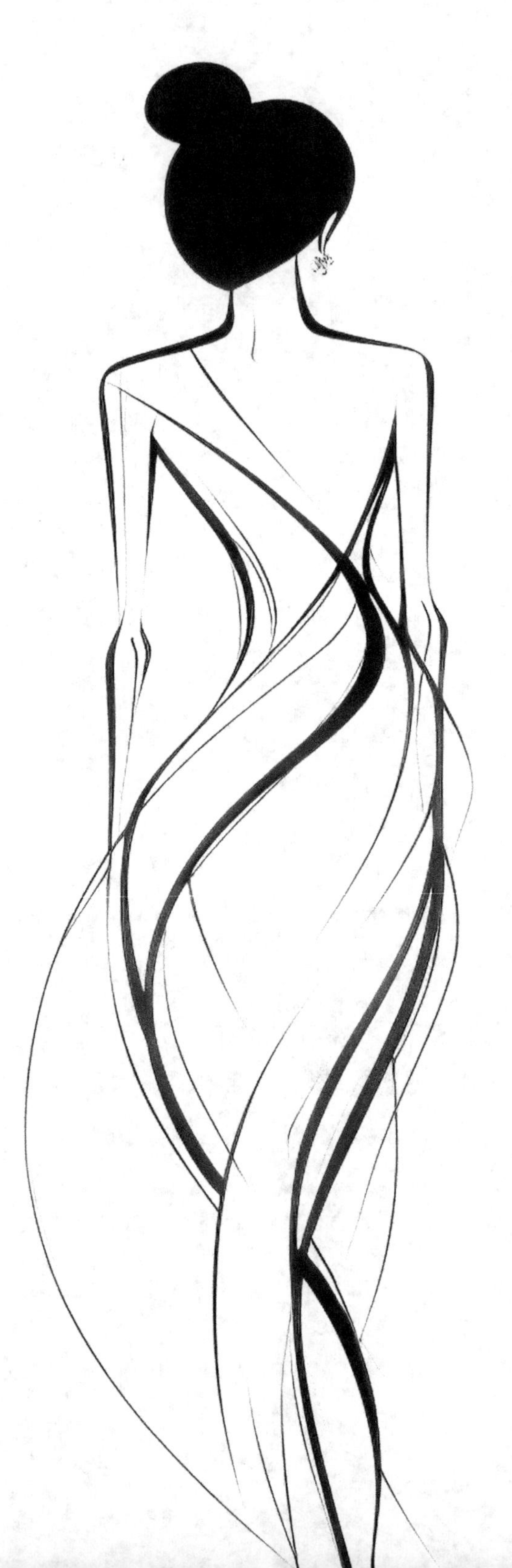

Chapter 14

Menopause Mayhem and Magic

*"We need a change
of heart, a reframing
of all our conceptions
and a new orientation
of our activities."* [1]

Letter on Behalf
of Shoghi Effendi

Over our lifetimes, women's bodies transition through several dramatic stages of development, following one from each other until we reach old age. Once we have navigated the growing pains of puberty, we may then go through pregnancy, birth and nursing raising children – and all the exhaustion and physical shape-shifting that entails. Once out of those years, we may have a brief respite before hitting perimenopause at any age from 35 – the stage leading up to the end of our reproductive years, called menopause. Then, finally, we reach post-menopause.

These life stages bring their joys but they take their toll as well. For my part, being pregnant or nursing three baby girls for nine years brought me so much peace and purpose, but it certainly put a strain on my physical body. It takes about a year after we stop nursing for our hormones to re-regulate to normal. My hormones didn't get back to balance until ten years after my missed menses with my first pregnancy. By then I was 38. I felt great in my late 30s and early 40s… until I hit 44 and I entered perimenopause: the stage lasting an average of seven to ten years leading up to our last menstrual cycle. Menopause is the 12-month period following that final menses; after that, we enter post-menopause.

Of all the life stages women go through, perimenopause is usually the most challenging. Perimenopause is the process when the production of sex hormones (estrogen, progesterone, and testosterone) by the ovaries gradually tapers off, as the adrenal glands begin to take over the production of these sex hormones instead. During early perimenopause, progesterone is often the first to begin to drop. And the more pregnancies and stress you have experienced, the lower the progesterone becomes. In late-stage perimenopause, estrogen suddenly declines.

During perimenopause, your hormones are at their most erratic as they fluctuate wildly. During this time, you may wake up feeling tired and exhausted one day and tearful and moody the next.

One minute you are full of zest, have mental clarity and a sense of wellbeing – then, without warning, the smallest trigger leads to anger, rage or a sense of depression and low self-esteem. When it all calms down, you find yourself apologetic and remorseful, telling yourself and perhaps those you reacted to, 'This is not me. I'm not sure what came over me! I am so sorry.'

What came over you was a 'hormone seizure' – when your body releases hormones in abrupt, irregular spurts while it attempts to re-establish balance as the sex hormones start to decline. When these hormone seizures strike without warning, your behaviors and your emotions may be unpredictable and your mood swings volatile. They are made worse because your stressed organs are unable to completely process the overload of toxins and hormones. Levels of blood sugar and insulin, adrenal stress hormones, thyroid hormones, and the function of your pituitary gland all become erratic and dysregulated. Your risk for pre-diabetes, heart disease, high cholesterol, fatigue, thyroid issues, and burnout multiplies, and your periods become irregular – anything from two ovulations a month to cycles more than 35 days apart or missed completely.

During perimenopause, some women may experience hot flashes, heart palpitations, mood anxiety, abdominal pain and gas, brain fog, sleep problems and even rashes and itching. These point to the dysregulation of the autonomic nervous system, because hormones are intricately linked to the autonomic nervous system through the neuro-endocrine system. When your neuro-endocrine system dysregulates, you may feel as though you are going crazy.

Negative thoughts, such as anger, depression, panic attacks and anxiety, add to the chaotic expression of the physical symptoms. The confusion and dysregulation of the autonomic nervous system creates instability, which may make you feel you cannot rely on your body or trust it. You may start to doubt yourself, your body, your purpose and direction in all aspects of life. You think to yourself – when will these challenges end?

Angelina Jolie, Gwyneth Paltrow and Michelle Obama are among the many celebrities who have started to open up about their experiences of perimenopause and menopause to help empower and educate other women going through the same rollercoaster ride, which has been a taboo for so long. So, how do we address these unpredictable symptoms that affect us at all levels: physically, mentally, emotionally, sexually and, perhaps, even spiritually? How do we try to regulate a hormonal process that is automatic and serves an essential function in our day-to-day life?

Unfortunately, there is no quick-fix solution for the challenges of this life experience. We are more likely to experience difficult rides through perimenopause, including more intense 'hormone seizures', when our lifestyle practices during the decades leading up to perimenopause have caused blood sugar dysregulation and burnout of our stress hormones. This is because when we enter perimenopause at a low ebb, with low adrenal gland reserves, our adrenal glands find it harder to take over the ovaries' role of producing the sex hormones.

Therefore, the more we do good for our body, mind, and spirit in our teens, 20s and 30s, the less likely we are to experience frequent and intense hormone seizures as we journey through perimenopause in our 40s and 50s. This means prioritizing regular exercise, good sleep hygiene, balanced work/life practices, healthy eating habits, reducing our exposure to toxins (such as smoking and alcohol), stress management techniques and positive self-talk. Spiritual practices of meditation and prayer and being of service to others reinforce these positive lifestyle choices.

If you are already in your 40s and 50s and experiencing intense hormone seizures, it is never too late to reframe your conceptions and shift your mindset, your lifestyle and spiritual practices and your nutrition. It will take work but it is worth it. You will feel happier, more youthful, and more vibrant while reducing your risks for chronic illness, heart disease, cancer and dementia. The choices and the shifts you make now will potentially minimize your risks for age-related long-term suffering and chronic disease.

Is Your Liver on Overload?

An overloaded liver can exacerbate the rollercoaster ride of perimenopause, because the basic role of the liver to process hormones and break them down into byproducts (called metabolites) to be eliminated through the bowels and urine becomes compromised, slower or stagnant. Some of you may have experienced intensified hot flashes or night sweats on the nights you consume alcohol, for example. Younger women may experience severe mood swings, bloating, or acne before menstruation. These symptoms often occur because the liver is depleted of glutathione and overloaded with toxins: anger and resentment, chemicals, glyphosate, alcohol, pollution, viruses, parasites, bacteria, and yeast.

We can reduce the stress on the liver by reducing the toxic exposure from our environment and lifestyle, calming our minds by processing anger and resentment, and nourishing the liver by providing it with nutrients including glutathione support, clean water, healthy blood and oxygen circulation, and good sleep. Once the stress on the liver is diminished, the liver processes the extra hormones produced during hormone seizures more efficiently. This helps stabilize the emotional and physical perimenopausal reactions while fostering total wellbeing.

Hormone Replacement Therapy: Good or Bad?

In addition to dietary and lifestyle modifications, when patients need support during perimenopause and menopause, I usually prescribe a combination of bioidentical E3 (estriol) and E2 (estradiol) hormones in a compounded cream form, called Biest.

When prescribed correctly and pulsed on and off, Biest transdermal cream re-establishes healthier estrogen levels in women, especially if started early during menopause, to improve symptoms and quality of life while lowering the risks of chronic disease such as dementia[2], heart disease[3] and osteoporosis[4]. Sometimes, I prescribe bioidentical E2 as a pellet inserted under the skin, with compounded E3 applied vaginally to support dry and thinning vaginal tissue and to help reduce risks of cancer and inflammation during menopause and post-menopause[5].

When the largest-ever study on hormone replacement therapy (HRT), the 2002 Women's Health Initiative trial[6], was stopped early because of increased risk of breast cancer and death from heart disease and stroke, fear among doctors and female patients about the risks of using HRT rose so significantly that it paralyzed the therapy's widespread use. What was not made clear in the media, however, was that the trials tested the use of synthetic hormone therapy, and not the safer bio-identical hormone therapy. The negative results were associated mostly with synthetic progestin.

Doctors stopped prescribing hormone therapy and women stopped using it. As a result, women in their perimenopause, menopause and post-menopausal years have unnecessarily suffered physically, mentally, and emotionally for over 20 years now. Since then, women's hormones (and, really, women's femininity and total health) have bottomed out, and not been supported as they should.

Many women in these age groups suffering with menopausal symptoms have been commonly told by their doctors, "You are depressed, and you need some anti-depressants," or they have been ignored and demoralized. Their male partners, at times, have regarded them as 'crazy', not understanding nor respecting how the changes in a women's body impact their behavior, mood, physical and mental health.

But women going through menopause are not deficient in Prozac or Lexapro. Menopausal women are deficient in estrogens and other hormones, which makes them anxious, moody and depressed. In the last decade, more studies have focused on the use and safety of bio-identical hormone replacement therapies (BHRT) and food to ease women's symptoms and improve their health outcomes.

From the vast amount of further research on BHRT in the last 20 years, for the sake of women's health and their relationships, sometimes it may be important for women to use some form of personalized bio-identical hormone therapy to improve mental health and mood, to reduce inflammation and the risk of heart disease and cancer, while also promoting brain and bone health and their general wellbeing. For some healthy women, the benefits of properly prescribed personalized bio-identical hormone therapy outweigh the risks of not using BHRT.

To make clear again, I am talking about bio-identical hormone therapy, which means hormone therapies that are plant-based, often derived from wild yams, and generally act in identical ways to one's biological hormones. Bio-identical hormones are different from synthetic hormone therapies, like Premarin or Provera, which influence the body very differently, potentially increasing inflammation and the risks of cancer, blood clots and heart disease. Bio-identical hormone therapy appears to be more efficacious and associated with lower risks of breast cancer and cardiovascular disease than synthetic hormone therapy. For now, studies consider BHRT to be the preferred form of hormone therapy[7].

When I reflect back to the last four decades of my life, I realize that I have put my body through a lot of stress, sometimes by choice and other times by circumstance, ultimately setting me up for lower adrenal reserves and liver overload. I had multiple childhood antibiotics and vaccinations, a mouth full of amalgams by age 10, then went from undergraduate work directly into naturopathic medical school. Training intensively in my 20s was followed by three pregnancies and nursing, then full-time practice, two fellowships and a board-certification – all without a break.

Now, as expected of a 54-year-old with lower adrenal reserves transitioning through menopause, I too have experienced hormone seizures – even though I follow a very clean diet, a conscious lifestyle and spiritual practices. How could I not, after using up all my reserves during the last four decades?

Thankfully, I am now so much more aware of my toxic exposures, positive thought processes, spiritual practices, eating and lifestyle habits and, of course, my hormone and nutrition support than I was in my 20s. My hormone seizures are relatively mild and under control.

Nevertheless, I have to stay constantly mindful of my thoughts, nutrition, toxic exposures and maintaining my exercise regime. This requires constant awareness and hard work but I feel elated, grounded, and with a strong sense of wellbeing and purpose as a result. I am grateful for how my body continues to perform youthfully to achieve my life's meaningful purpose.

So, the good news is that even though perimenopause may be very difficult for many due to the modern-day stressors imposed on women, postmenopause – the 12 months after the final menses – is often much less dramatic than perimenopause. In fact, many of my female patients report that the two years after menopause are the best of their lives. Libido, energy, memory, vitality, skin quality, physical strength and general outlook on life appear to be optimum during the post-menopausal years, if the body, mind and spirit are regularly depurated while supported with personalized BHRT, good nutrition, sleep, meditation, prayer and positive acts of service.

So, if you are in perimenopause and are having a hard time, remember that your best years are soon to be experienced. Stay patient, resilient and positive. Do your work and reach out for naturopathic hormone support... you are almost there!

Menopause is an opportunity for growth, for gratitude, for honor, for rebirth. It is an opportunity to sit with our spirit and soul, to meditate, reflect, and exercise our spiritual connection, to realign ourselves. It gives us the opportunity to be grateful for what we have experienced so far, for what our ancestors have taught us, and for all we have learnt.

Think of it as an opening for you to do things differently, to build new essential relationships, to be at one with your Creator and to carry forward what the generations of women who came before you began. We have an opportunity to rise to higher frequencies, to elevate ourselves to live a more powerful and transformative life. Though age is a number, expanding yourself to feel beyond the cultural inferences that number poses can be freeing. A positive mindset around aging potentially slows down your biological age (we will discuss this further in a later chapter).

After going through perimenopause, menopause and finally reaching post-menopause while simultaneously reaching the height of her career, Oprah Winfrey explained: "This is the moment to reinvent yourself after focusing on the needs of everyone else."

The Gen X Menopause Challenge

My generation of Gen X women grew up in the 1970s and 1980s, when many mothers had entered the workforce. We learned at an early age how to stand on our own two feet and navigate life's challenges without relying on others. Thanks to these cultural circumstances, most Gen X's are independent, resourceful, hard-working and adept problem-solvers.

But it goes a little further than that for Gen X women. As we became adults, we told ourselves we must do it all and do it with excellence: be the best wife, mother, daughter and friend, have accomplished careers, look good, create a beautiful home, raise fantastic children, take care of our elderly parents well – the tick-list never ends.

Many of us did accomplish all that and more – until we got to our forties and fifties and we now realize we are burnt out and exhausted. Many of us are sandwiched between caring for aging parents while simultaneously raising our own teenagers, working full careers, becoming empty nesters, attending to our partners, and then going through perimenopause or menopause during a post-traumatic global pandemic. Now we are in menopause: still exhausted, lacking vitality and libido, and suffering from stiff joints, weight gain, sleepless nights, forgetfulness and lack of self-esteem. What's to come next?

Interestingly, the chronic stress that the majority of us perimeno-pausal/menopausal Gen X women experienced, and continue to experience, has forced us to rethink who we are, to learn new ways of being, to re-evaluate our priorities and relationships, and to let go of the expectations, toxins and baggage (physical, emotional, mental and environmental) that we have clung to for decades.

We have had to re-evaluate our careers and our purpose. Forces are directing us to rise to higher heights, to become even more resilient as we lead ourselves, our children and the next generations towards creating a world that is more unified, instilling within it more feminine qualities of compassion, understanding, acceptance, kindness and gentleness.

In a sense, the pandemic forced many of us Gen X women to explore how we can create alignment with the Greater Good. What do we need to do to re-establish vitality, energy, elation and peace within ourselves so we can be vehicles of transformation for others? How can we continue to help shift the planet towards a more united and peaceful society? How do we strengthen our inner vitality and achieve our purpose? How do we create community that serves us all positively?

I wish I had an easy response to these questions, but I don't. Each one of us has a unique and individualized path, a blueprint to explore and grow through. It takes hard work and conscious effort to examine how our habits, thoughts, lifestyle practices and choices have led us to our current state – and then working out how to let them go and transform to a new way of conscious being - individually and collectively.

Virtue III

The KHOSH Method™

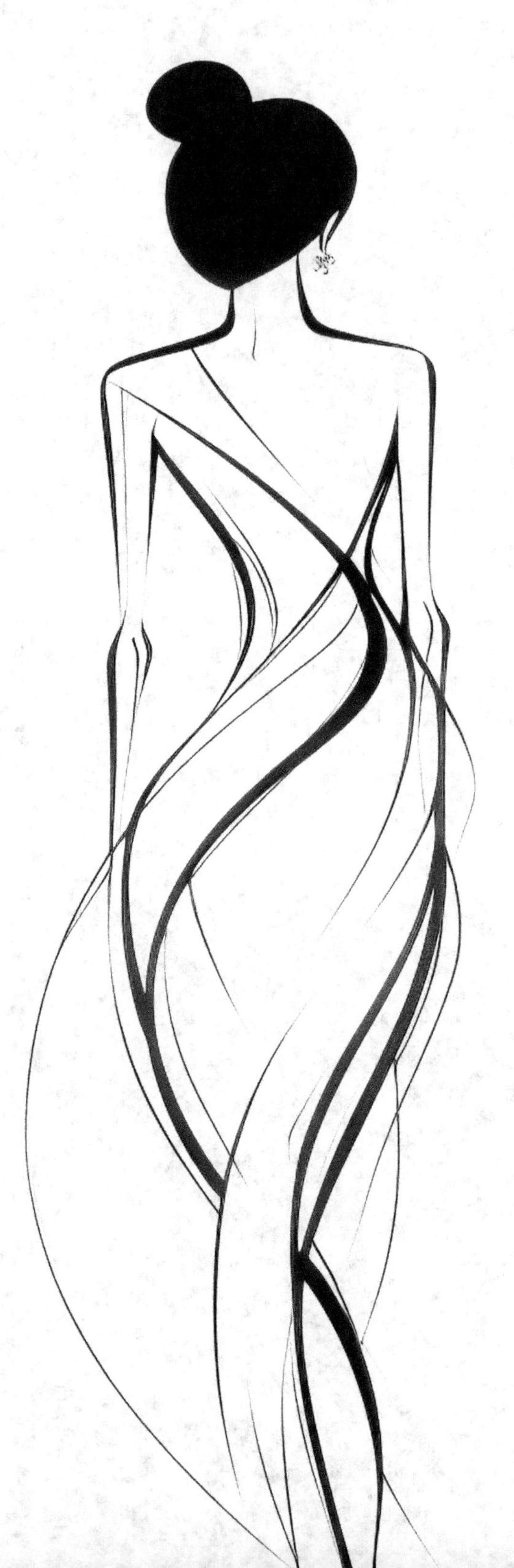

Chapter 15

Why We Age

"There is a fountain of youth: it is your mind, your talents, the creativity you bring to your life and the lives of the people you love. When you learn to tap this source, you will truly have defeated age."

Sophia Loren

I remember as a child looking up to my 50-year-old aunt and thinking she was old. But now I am in my fifties, I do not consider myself old and my friends and patients often see me as younger than I am. And yet, I see patients and friends in their forties who believe they are old.

The way we age partly depends on our how we perceive ourselves moving through life. If we believe we are old, we get old. When older people maintain a younger mindset, they age slower physically[1]. A study by Ellen Langer asked a group of people over 75 to live the way they did in their twenties – such as listening to the music of their youth and dressing like their 20-something selves[2]. After a week, photos and blood tests showed their faces looked younger and their inflammatory blood markers had significantly improved. Becoming ageless means freeing ourselves from the physical and mental constrictive boundaries we have set for ourselves, and instead soaring into the realm of the soul, the spirit. Here we can attain a boundless mindset and an ageless mind and body.

To understand how we can slow – and perhaps even reverse – aging from a physiological perspective, we must first understand some of the reasons behind aging and then begin to address each process in turn to regain youthfulness. Intuitively, we all know stress is the main reason we age. Mental, physical, emotional and environmental stressors create inflammation which leads to a host of other physiological problems in the body, including shortening cellular life (see the diagram on The Aging Process on the next page).

However, we have the capacity to shift our perception of stressful events and situations to reduce the stress in our cells, using the techniques I will explain in this section. As we do so, we increase joy and improve our wellbeing and longevity.

The Aging Process

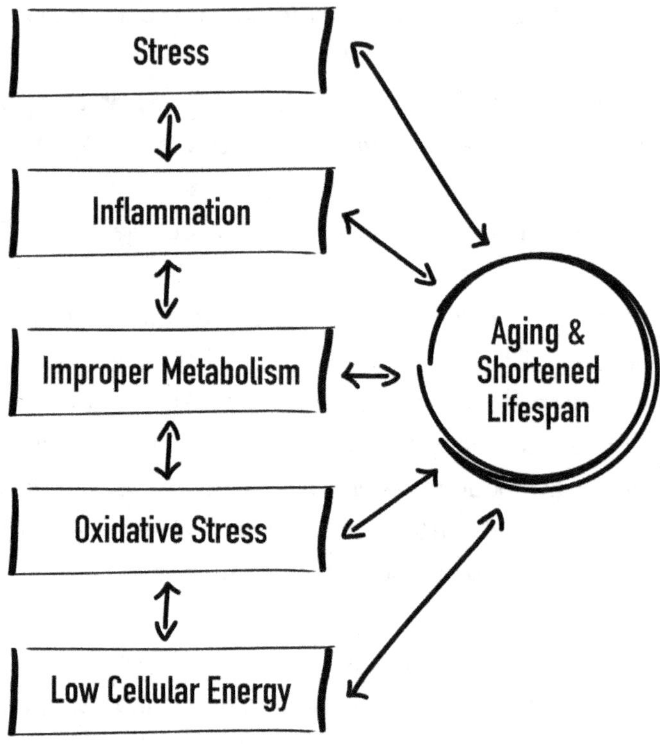

Our emotional and spiritual states affect how we age just as much as our physiological processes. In fact, even perceived stress – either what we perceive to be stressful, or remember to be stressful – activates multiple cellular mechanisms that cause aging, including inflammation, metabolism problems, oxidative stress and lower energy production. Your body and brain cannot tell the difference between an event that happened this morning and something that happened decades ago. You can be triggered into the stress response when a word, a smell, a comment, a picture or a song reminds your subconscious of the traumatic event of decades past. Immediately, your body goes into an intense reaction of pain and depression.

If you can shift your perspective of a traumatic experience and find the positivity within it – the learning and growth it enabled – while re-teaching your autonomic nervous system to respond to that memory or thought differently, you can potentially shift the stress response in your cells and slow the aging process. Think back to a stressful experience. Can you shift your perspective to see things from a positive space? Can you disconnect your memory from your physiological bodily reactions?

Although the process of shifting memories from trauma to a neutral or even positive state can be difficult, techniques such as meditation, EMDR (eye movement desensitization reprocessing), EFT (Emotional Freedom Technique), brain-spotting, ND Square™ and NAET (Nambudripad Allergy Elimination Technique) can help you dissociate the traumatic memory from your physiological stress response and cellular memory. It takes time and it takes work – consistent work. But once you have successfully dissociated a traumatic memory from your bodily experience and autonomic nervous response, you will find it difficult to even remember the experience fully and there will be no feeling attached to it.

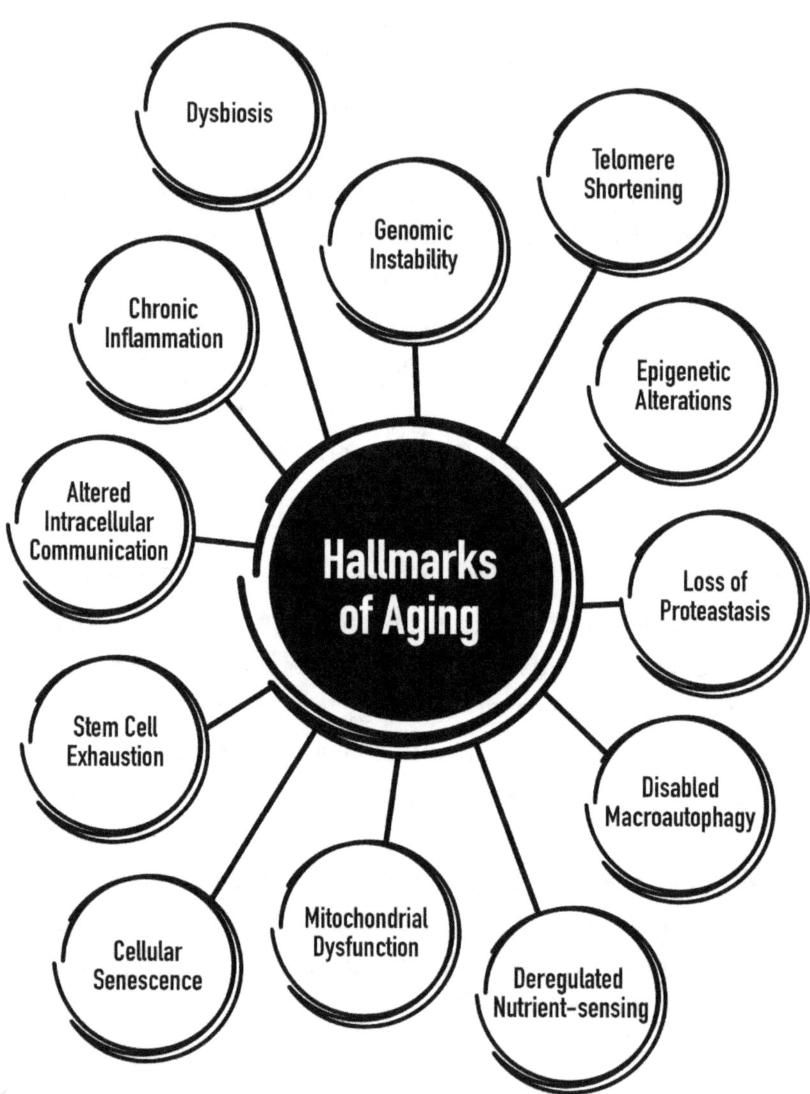

The diagram above shows 12 major internal physiological hallmarks behind aging[3]. DNA breaks down as we age, and its slow repair is central to the aging process. When either internal or external toxins cause our cells' DNA to break down, this triggers cell mutations, as well as the signals that cause our DNA to repair.

The seesaw between its breakdown and repair must be kept in constant balance to slow aging[4]. It is beyond the scope of this book to explain each of the physiological reasons for aging in scientific detail. Nevertheless, I will point out some of the more notable ones: mitochondrial health, genomic (DNA) stability, senescent cells, oxidative stress, protein homeostasis loss, telomere shortening, dysbiosis, and stem cell exhaustion. For further explanations, see my website **GoldenGateBook.com/resources.**

Cellular Senescence

Senescence, a major hallmark of aging, technically refers to a dynamic process of permanent cell cycle arrest in response to acute or chronic damage[5]. Senescent cells – such as dry skin that sloughs off after sunburn – no longer divide and duplicate in response to either external or internal stimuli. Aging results when senescent cells accumulate and the body cannot clean them up efficiently.

Mitochondria Dysfunction

The health of our mitochondria – the engines of our cells – must be maintained for as long as possible to slow aging. Aging occurs when the mitochondria are damaged by factors such as estrogen deficiency, oxidative stress or genetic mutations. When the mitochondria are not functioning as they should, the first symptoms commonly include fatigue, weight gain, brain fog and sleep problems, all of which indicate aging. When the mitochondria have not been properly functioning for years, chronic aging diseases such as Parkinson's, Alzheimer's, diabetes and cancer often set in.

Oxidative Stress and Inflammaging

Oxygen is vital to our cells' survival because it feeds the fire within us – but it also leaves behind ash, which is constantly swept up by our body's anti-oxidant system. When there are not enough sweepers (antioxidants) to clean up the ash, the ash that sticks around makes cells sick, damaged and inflamed. Age-related processes causing chronic cellular damage and inflammation leading to aging are known as inflammaging. Foods high in antioxidants reduce inflammaging and slow aging because they boost mitophagy (cellular cleaning up of dead mitochondria) and autophagy (cellular cleaning up of dead cells). Antioxidants basically exfoliate your insides.

Protein Homeostasis Loss

Proteins are vital to our physical life because they are involved in all our body's functions, including our genetics, hormones, muscles, and immune system. When the balance between these protein functions breaks down, we call it proteostasis, which is a sign of aging.

Instability

The health of our DNA and its ability to repair itself plays a major role in aging. When our DNA is damaged by internal and external toxins, the integrity of the genome is compromised. This leads to the build-up of senescent cells and can induce neurodegenerative conditions, cancer and age-related diseases. We can support genomic stability by prolonged exercise and intermittent fasting[6].

Telomere Shortening

The protective tips of our DNA are called telomeres (a form of bodyguard) – and they shorten when the cells are damaged. The shortened bodyguards provide less protection and make the DNA more unstable. The longer the telomeres, the slower the aging. Chinese herbs such as Centella asiatica[7] and oleanic acid (from olive oil) have been shown to protect telomere length[8]. Flavonoids such as quercetin, found in the yellow pigment of onions, and curcumin, an extract from the spice turmeric, can protect mitochondria and DNA from oxidative stress and damage[9]. Quercetin and curcumin are among foods that also activate AMPK, a cellular energy-boosting enzyme that regulates cell growth, metabolism and autophagy[10,11].

Dysbiosis

As you learnt in Chapter 11, the gut is the grand central station to everything in the body, including healthy aging. When the gut microbiome is imbalanced, known as dysbiosis, inflammation increases. A healthy microbiome has a balance between pro-inflammatory and anti-inflammatory bacteria, plus bacteria that produce short-chain fatty acids, like butyrate[12]. The healthier the microbiome, the lower the inflammation, the calmer the nervous system, the more balanced your estrogen levels, and the stronger your immune function and emotional health. In other words, the healthier the gut, the more gracefully you age.

Stem Cell Exhaustion

Stem cells are like the seeds your body uses to grow different types of cells, like bone, nerve, blood, fat and muscle cells. When stem cells are depleted, tissues and cells cannot repair themselves or regenerate efficiently and aging sets in. This is known as stem cell exhaustion. For tips on therapies that can enhance the function of your stem cells – and even, in some cases, reverse the aging process – please see my book website, GoldenGateBook.com/resources.

Be Joyful ('Khosh Baash')

Khosh, which means "joy" in Farsi, my mother tongue, and is the first part of my maiden name, Khoshkhesal, is the final destination for all of us. The next world is thought to consist of only joy. I believe if we can achieve true joy in this world of existence, we can feel, look and be more youthful – in short, our psychological sense of joy and wellbeing[13] can potentially slow and possibly reverse the aging process.

Joy, or khosh, is the most elevated emotion we humans experience. It creates wellbeing, encompassing mental, spiritual and physical health. Joy and love both resonate at the frequency of 528 Hz. This particular frequency is the vibration of nature, of chlorophyll in plants. In his book *The Book of 528: Prosperity Key of Love*, the Harvard scholar Dr. Leonard G Horowitz proved this frequency to be the Universal Healer. He says this frequency is required for space/time measurements; it gives rise to circles, squares, arches and architecture; it is needed to determine the speed of light; and it is paramount to the structure of water and hemoglobin.

For centuries, it has been thought that listening to music at the frequency of 528 Hz elevates the soul and heals the body. In the musical scale Do-Re-Mi-Fa-So-La-Si-Do, 'Mi' or the note 'E', resonates at 528 Hz. Historically, this frequency was known as the 'miracle tone' in the Solfeggio frequencies: a set of six tones based on ancient Gregorian chants. It was used by Gregorian monks for its powerful healing, restorative and transformative properties. The John Lennon song *Imagine* generally resonates at 528 Hz and is soothing to the nervous system. So, too, do the Beatles hit *Hey Jude* and songs by Bob Marley and Pink Floyd.

In the 1970s, the mathematician and physician Dr. Joseph Puleo rediscovered the extraordinary benefits of the Solfeggio frequencies, mathematically linking 528 Hz to restorative healing. It has been theorized that this frequency can stimulate transformation and heal DNA. A study on rats showed that it appeared to reverse cell damage caused by reactive oxidative species (ROS) in the brain, which is produced by the body in response to stress and toxins. In the same rat study, the 528 Hz frequency decreased P450 aromatase gene expression in rats' brains, which means improved detoxification of estrogens, while inducing increase testosterone production[14].

Through the science of bi-directional psychoneurophysiology, we are learning that positive emotions impact our physical, mental and social health, and our spirituality and aging[15]. Positive thoughts improve the gut microbiome, which leads to healthier immune function and physical and mental wellbeing. Joy, for instance, potentially reverses the main hallmarks of aging such as lowering inflammation, supporting mitochondrial health, correcting microbiome disruptions, and other aging mechanisms in cells while elevating your spirit and soul[16].

Joy can also influence your physical appearance, making you look younger[17]. The reciprocal relationship also holds true: as you take care of your health, appearance and relationships, your optimism and joy increase – especially in the more senior years[18]. It is a positive feedback system: be joyful to age youthfully, and take care of your health, your appearance and your relationships to create more joy[19]. Being creative also promotes joy. See what happens to your wellbeing when you are creative in the way you approach your daily life, your relationships, your work and your purpose.

Now you understand why khosh is so important in youthful aging, and the wisdom behind my mother's frequent advice to me "be joyful" ("khosh baash"). After decades of hearing "khosh baash" from my mother during challenging times, I finally realized the wisdom she was sharing with me for my own wellbeing and longevity. Using a systematic approach, my KHOSH Method™ aims to help you restore your wellbeing, elevate your sense of health to regenerate your cells, mind and spirit, and increase joy within your cells.

I personally practice the KHOSH Method™ on a daily basis and have taught many of my patients to do the same. Though you will learn the basics of the KHOSH Method™ in this book, I encourage you to access my website, **GoldenGateBook.com/resources**, as I delve deeper into the practical details of the KHOSH Method™, revealing more of my secrets to youthful aging.

So, over the following chapters, let's explore the six-step approach of the KHOSH Method™ to achieve your joy and total wellbeing. Keep in mind that in order for the method to help you regain and maintain your health and slow the aging process, you must consistently do your work, make mindful choices, and practice awareness, faith, love, patience and persistence.

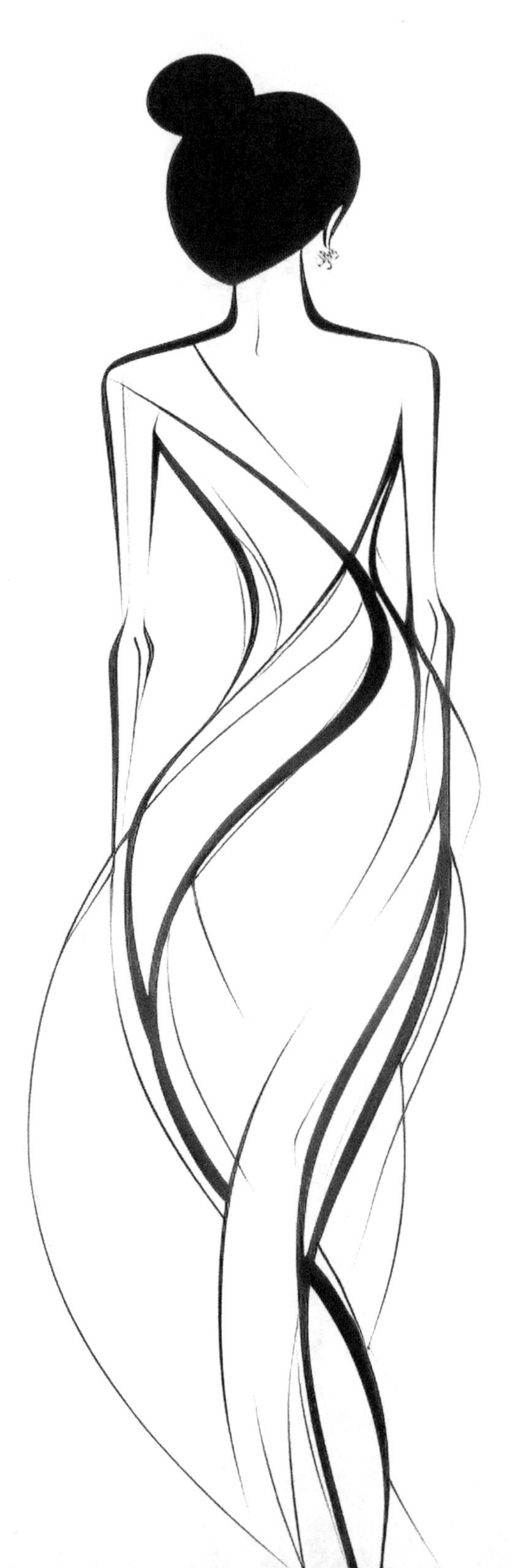

Chapter 16

Six Steps to Graceful Aging

"*I want you to be happy…
to laugh, smile
and rejoice in order
that others may be
made happy by you.*"

Annamarie Honnold,
Vignettes from the Life
of 'Abdu'l-Bahá

The KHOSH Method™ is a simple six-step process to unleash your feminine powers towards graceful aging, to joyfulness, to your life's meaningful purpose and the happiness you deserve. The method will bring you meaningful joy and help you lead a transformative, youthful life so you can be an agent of positive change for the world around you.

The KHOSH Method™ involves addressing the wellbeing of the Five Gems of Longevity™ within you: the spiritual, physical, mental, emotional and social/community. Each Gem affects the other and they are all interrelated, so skipping over one Gem potentially causes health risks and jeopardizes your longevity. For example, working only on your spiritual health while ignoring your physical health and your relationships will create stress in another part of your wellbeing, hence compromising your longevity. And focusing on your physical health while ignoring the other Gems will create distress in the system. The Five Gems illustrated in the diagram on the following page must be kept in balance and unity for health, longevity, and joy.

As you move through each of the six steps of the KHOSH Method™, make sure to address the Five Gems at each level. This will ensure a more thorough approach to healing and elevating all aspects of yourself. The diagram on the next page identifies the Five Gems and some of the aspects of each Gem that you must mindfully choose to address, heal, acknowledge and practice regularly to strengthen that Gem.

The Five Gems of Longevity

The six steps are listed in the next diagram. I will delve into each step in more detail on the book's website, GoldenGateBook.com/resources, but for now, remember these six steps in order and work on activating each one. You may think about working on the first step for a month or so as a start, and then adding in the next step for the next month or so. Be mindful that these steps are not necessarily linear, and some people may need to move through them synergistically and simultaneously.

The KHOSH Method™: Six Steps to Graceful Aging

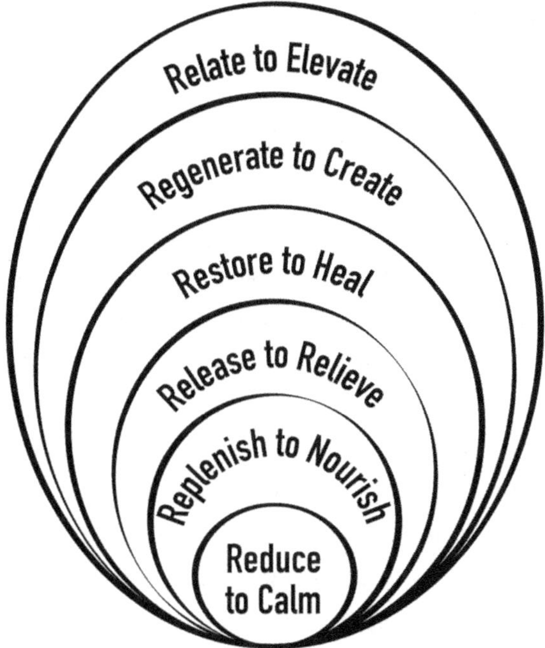

These steps will need to be cycled through a few times as you discover more root cause imbalances and strive to clear, correct, balance and heal them. You may find you circle through steps three and four a few times, especially if you are in perimenopause or menopause. Each time you will delve deeper into layers of your cellular and subconscious you were not aware of in the past, but which were hidden blocks to your healing. I think of it like a corkscrew effect. Each time you work through steps three and four, you are screwing your corkscrew deeper into the cellular, energetic and spiritual realms and becoming more aware, more refined, more clear, more elevated.

Once you have worked through all six steps at least once, you may need to go through the steps again, especially as life throws curve balls, like the COVID-19 pandemic. Those who had already moved through the six steps often found themselves stronger and more resilient to be able to handle COVID-19 and the pandemic. And those who were stuck on the first floor, severely inflamed, found it difficult to move to the next steps.

Think about these six steps as steps of a floor in a high-rise building. You have many floors to go through as you move through life. Each time it becomes easier to go up the next floor as you are no longer carrying the heavy baggage of the past – your weight is lighter – though the steepness may be more challenging as you rise to higher heights. With every floor, you are able to be more present, more conscious, and have increased capacity to achieve greater heights, especially spiritually.

After completing at least one round of the six steps, you may want to create a daily maintenance program with your physician, where you incorporate regular lifestyle practices, nutrition, habits and spiritual exercises at each step throughout each day, week or month. At the end of each day, bring yourself to account, give yourself love and gratitude, and focus on positivity for the next day.

Remember that the KHOSH Method™ and any information contained in this book is not to be substituted for any medical advice for your particular condition. Please consult your licensed physician or reach out to me at **https://drdarvish.com/** to receive personalized medical support during your health journey. Remember the information presented in this book is for educational purposes only.

Step 1:

Reduce to Calm

> *"Within you,
> there is a stillness
> and a sanctuary
> to which you can
> retreat at any time
> and be yourself."*

Hermann Hesse

Modern lifestyle stressors signal the body's inflammatory response to protect and save itself from hazard. It is like calling 911 and activating the emergency response. Examples of these stressors include your diet and the quality of the food you eat, your electromagnetic and cellular exposure, environmental and dental toxins, infections, and mental thoughts.

The processes activating your immune system response to clean up these toxins cause inflammation. The gut becomes inflamed and the microbiome disturbed. The brain fogs up. Energy slows. Hormones dysregulate. The autonomic nervous system goes chaotic. Depression or anxiety sets in. Sleep gets disrupted and pain signals fire. Pro-inflammatory chemicals, known as cytokines, travel to tissues promoting further inflammation leading to inflammaging. As we learned in previous chapters, stress provides the breeding ground for aging. It induces inflammation and the development of chronic disease, depression, metabolic disease, cardiovascular disease, immune deficiency, hormonal imbalances, and so much more[1].

Chronic inflammation reduces absorption of nutrients, disturbs hormones, increases toxicity of the matrix and creates generalized distress within the nervous system, among other systems. Reducing inflammation and stress thus provides an entry way to healing and youthful aging.

Therefore, the first step of the KHOSH Method™ is to calm the 'emergency response' by reducing inflammation and reducing exposure to everything you have control over: food allergies and sensitivities, artificial sweeteners, alcohol, food coloring and preservatives, recreational drugs, over-the-counter medications, electromagnetic fields and cell phones, heavy metals, chemicals, pesticides, tap-water, mold exposure, emotional stressors, long working hours, negative people and your own negative thoughts, for instance. Most importantly, avoid your exposure to backbiting and gossip, for they are the greatest evils of our modern life.

When you reduce toxic exposures, stress and inflammation, you give your cells, your mind, body and spirit, an opportunity for healing. You welcome your natural healing capacity to do their work. You welcome nature. You welcome art. You welcome joy! As the 16th century Swiss physician Paracelsus said: "The art of healing comes from nature, not from the physician. Therefore, the physician must start from nature, with an open mind."

You have the capacity to identify many of the initiators of dysfunction by becoming aware, by spiritually aligning yourself. Listen to your inner voice and practice detachment. The 'knowing' is within you. You know that the sugar you are eating or the wine you are drinking is only covering up suppressed deeper emotions, for example. What you may need is encouragement, discipline and love to reduce what no longer benefits your health, your wellbeing, your longevity.

You may want to start by reducing foods that you know are unhealthy and those foods which you know you are sensitive to. As Hippocrates' famous quote says: "Let food be thy medicine and medicine thy food." You want to make sure you are eating clean, organic foods void of processing, preservatives, artificial sweeteners and chemicals. Incorporating an anti-inflammatory plant-based diet (see Appendix A) is the vital first step in breaking the inflammatory cycle, because calming inflammation allows better absorption of nourishment. It is a virtuous circle, because calming inflammation calms the nervous system – and calming the nervous system helps calm inflammation.

I often like to start the day with gluten-free miso soup with mushrooms and organic sprouted tofu, especially in the winter months because of its incredible nourishing benefits, particularly during menopause or during the first half of the menstrual cycle[2]. Chia pudding with flaxseeds, hemp seeds, turmeric, cinnamon, cardamom and Himalayan salt in organic plant-based milk can be an alternative in warmer seasons.

Although an anti-inflammatory diet may initially appear restrictive, it is usually observed for a short period of four to six weeks, which is often achievable and can make much difference in reducing your inflammation and pain while helping you recognize your resilience and innate capacity for discipline. This diet often provides an opportune step to show kindness to yourself, to explore your strength, and to learn the healing effects of patience for yourself.

During this step, make sure you reduce exposure to toxins that affect all the Five Gems of Longevity, as set out earlier in this chapter. See Appendix A for the KHOSH Anti-Inflammatory Diet, different hydrotherapy tools, and plant-based anti-inflammatory supplements that may be used to reduce inflammation as part of this first step. You may want to set up a consultation with me or one of my colleagues to help you identify the substances that are seen by your particular system as inflammatory or toxic, which should be avoided during this first step.

Step 2:

Replenish to Nourish

"I am your moon and your
moonlight too
I am your flower garden
and your water too
I have come all this way,
eager for you
Without shoes or shawl
I want you to laugh
To kill all your worries
To love you
To nourish you."

Rumi

The birth of my firstborn was traumatic – both for me, and for my daughter. She suffered through a long 28 hours of labor and was stuck in the birth canal for hours. Finally, when she was pulled out by forceps, her neck had been strained and her head hurt. Because of the neck and head pain, she had trouble being held and nursed and she started to lose weight.

I was scared. I strongly believed my daughter would recover if I found a way to feed her, hold her, and nourish her. I prayed and meditated to ask for assistance for her healing. My mom and husband were there to help me, and friends came by to offer support and bring food and love.

Soon I figured out how to nourish her. I learned how to hold her so she would not experience pain but felt my love instead. Every hour for the first month of her life, while trying to recover from an intense traumatic birth myself, I would either nurse her or pump milk to feed her. Within a month, her weight turned around. She was sleeping through the night and her pain resolved. That experience taught me the importance of nourishment – physical, emotional, spiritual and from the community.

So, the second step in revolutionizing your health consists of replenishment and nourishment. Nourishing your Five Gems of Longevity with all they need provides the basis for your transformative process. The people you surround yourself with, the work you do, the books you read, the media you watch, the food you eat, the music you listen to, the air you breathe, the thoughts you think, and the community you engage with are all forms of nourishment or toxicity. They will either nourish you to live your best joyful and youthful life, or they will limit you towards fulfilling that destiny. You choose.

For a newborn to survive and thrive, the baby first requires nourishment at multiple levels: milk, physical touch, parental connection, sleep, warmth, trust, love and joy. Research has shown that even when an infant is nourished with food but is deprived of parental connection, for example, the baby fails to thrive[3]. The same holds true for us adults: we also need nourishment to thrive, but as adults we must provide nourishment for ourselves rather than relying on others.

Nourishment comes in different forms. Replenishing your cells with hydration, oxygen, nutrients, minerals, amino acids and healthy fats provides the fundamental building blocks for cellular and tissue healing and regeneration. But beyond consuming healthy organic whole foods, drinking clean water, breathing fresh air, exercising, and filling your heart and soul with love, you can gain courage and inner strength to move through the transformative process by building community and giving and receiving love.

Remember one of my favorite quotes by Baha'u'llah: "Love Me that I may love thee. If thou lovest Me not, My love can in no wise reach thee.[4]" During this second step of my method, it is vital to build and strengthen relationships with those you trust, the ones you love, and with yourself. Connect to your Creator, to the Greater Good, to your living loved ones, and to your ancestors – for instance, through prayer, meditation and visualization. Smile and hug people daily: work up to at least 12 hugs per day for growth as psychotherapist Virginia Satir has said. Work on building a loving and supportive community around you. Most women subconsciously deprive themselves of nourishment, so learn to accept and receive nourishment. Without it, all the other steps in the KHOSH Method™ do not work as well.

In this step, make sure you are eating three meals per day with two snacks. Your meals should be organic as much as possible, comprising mostly plant-based whole foods that are easy to digest. Start with warm or cooked food to help you digest it easily. Drink room temperature filtered water, get sufficient regular sleep, think positively, exercise regularly, get fresh air, and create positive environments, relationships and community by emanating loving-kindness, trustworthiness, integrity, patience, compassion, empathy, love and joyfulness. When you are kind, you attract kindness and when you are resentful, you attract anger. Focus on being positive and loving with yourself and others to grow more love and positivity around you.

When you experience uncontrollable hormone seizures during perimenopause and menopause, your refuge and place to start to heal is to control the things you can control to offset the inflammatory reactions of the imbalanced hormones. Focus on replenishment and nourishment. If you are alone, perhaps get a pet – a dog, a cat. Find ways of filling your cup with goodness, with love and support. When you have nourished your Five Gems, you gain the strength to move through the next steps of the KHOSH Method™. You will find examples of methods to replenish to nourish yourself in Appendix B.

One of the best ways to protect yourself against aging, age-related frailty and sarcopenia (the loss of muscle as we age) while unleashing your feminine powers as you journey through life is to engage in physical activity and moderate exercise. Exercise, especially resistance exercise, builds muscle and bone while supporting the insulin-blood sugar balance[5]. Exercise helps support healthy hormones and nourishes your mind, body and spirit.

Muscle has more oxygen than fat. Fat generally collects chemicals, metals and toxins and promotes inflammation and aging in the body, while oxygen supports immune health and brain and heart health while reducing inflammation. Therefore, when muscle is replaced by fat as we age, or sarcopenia, we acquire more toxic build-up as a result of increased body fat and reduced oxygen levels, and our muscle mass and strength declines. Sarcopenia often sets in during perimenopause and menopause, when estrogen levels drop and inflammation increases. During menopause, metabolic syndrome and visceral fat – that spare tire around your belly – also increase as estrogen declines and cortisol, the stress hormone, activates.

The good news is that resistance exercise can fight against all of that[6]. My general recommendation, based on research given to my healthy female patients, is to do 15 to 20 minutes of strength/resistance exercises three to four times per week, combined with 20 to 30 minutes of mild/moderate aerobics five days per week. This provides a good balance of exercises to support the anti-aging and health benefits of exercise.

If you are menopausal or postmenopausal, make sure to have your estrogen levels evaluated and addressed. You may also want to take creatine supplements to optimize the benefits of exercise training and your energy levels – especially during menstruation, menopause or postmenopausal. Remember, the idea is not to become the next Olympian but to help unleash your feminine powers to create a healthy physique and to empower your mind and spirit so you can continue to be an agent of transformation. Again, it's best to consult your physician for the appropriate exercise program tailored to your particular health situation.

Hormones are Nourishing

Hormones are nourishing to us, but we often forget the importance of hormone balance and function in maintaining our health. A teenager needs her hormones to grow bones, muscles, mental capacity and immune function and capacity. When hormones are out of balance or depleted, they slow our capacity for growth, strength and stable mood.

During step two, hormones need to be evaluated and addressed. I use the DUTCH hormone urine and saliva test, along with blood tests, to identify the imbalance within the hormone cascades. I then support their production and metabolism by prioritizing an individualized food regime, healthy fats, herbs, nutrients and lifestyle practices – something you would discuss with your licensed naturopathic physician. When hormones are greatly depleted, sometimes bioidentical hormone therapy becomes essential.

For example, when muscles are weak, energy is low, and you are feeling ungrounded and indecisive, you may have low testosterone levels that need to be activated through diet, exercise, peptide therapy or testosterone replacement therapy. If you are stressed and on fight-and-flight response, you may need supportive therapies for the adrenal glands and the HPA (hypothalamus-pituitary-adrenal) axis, as well as the autonomic nervous system. Acupuncture, Ondamed biofeedback therapy, body work, homeopathy, meditation, diet manipulation and herbal medicine are some techniques that may help nourish your adrenals and the HPA axis.

If I plan to prescribe personalized bio-identical hormone therapy, I make sure that Step three is optimized first. I need to make sure that the liver is efficiently detoxifying toxic hormones before I add an extra hormone load to the liver. If your liver is not metabolizing hormones properly, I do not want to increase your risk of hormone-related cancers and inflammation. In this instance, we wait to start bio-identical hormone replacement therapy until Step three has been optimized.

Beyond Physical Nourishment

During late perimenopause, when my stress levels were extraordinarily high due to my parents dying, moving homes, becoming an empty nester, shifts in our staff and the COVID-19 pandemic, I began experiencing chronic hives – a histamine response to the changes in hormones and the intense stress. Instead of experiencing hot flashes, I would experience hives and angioedema (allergic swelling of the face and lips). I tried everything to calm the hives, but nothing worked.

You could say I was not my joyful self. I felt guilty that I was not practicing my mom's wish for me to be joyful. I began to visualize my mother and father holding me, talking to me, showing me their love, and advising me. I began talking to their souls and I felt their love once again. I finally allowed myself to feel the grief and the pain of losing all that had been in the past, and mindfully choosing to see the opportunities of the present – to recognize new possibilities for building a more joyful future. I intensified my prayer, meditation, visualization and emotional clearing practice and I started Ondamed biofeedback therapy, acupuncture and reflexology – they calmed my nerves and reset my nervous system response.

Through prayer and meditation and being patient with myself, I learnt to accept nourishment and love from the Universe. I released the deeply seated fight-and-flight response engraved within my cells from generational trauma. I finally accepted the new path I was being guided to – one that was to be more powerful, more revolutionary and more joyful than I had ever been before. The hives calmed and my hormones reorganized themselves. I am now stronger, more resilient and healthier. I feel more joyful and function with youthful vitality again.

In this second step of the KHOSH Method™, physical nourishment by itself is often insufficient to support thriving health. We need emotional nourishment through touch, connecting with others, building strong relationship bonds and engaging in community. We also need to nourish our mental and intellectual wellbeing through learning something new on a daily basis, such as solving puzzles, reading, playing an instrument, learning a new dance routine and writing. Daily practice of creativity nourishes our mental and emotional wellbeing.

Since we are spiritual beings journeying this world in a physical body, we must also fuel our soul if we want to thrive. Ways to nourish your soul are practicing gratitude; showing respect, compassion, kindness, love, and wisdom to ourselves and others; and praying, meditating and reflecting on a daily basis. Soulful music, elevated authentic conversations, sound baths, time in nature, or creative play with babies are other ways to fuel your soul.

When we fuel our soul, our thoughts become more embracing, our minds more loving, our perspectives more adaptable, and our perceived stressors are reduced – all of which inhibit the fight-and-flight response and shift our nervous system towards the healing parasympathetic response. Ultimately, the healing and regenerative systems within our cells are activated while our soul elevates to a higher frequency of joy. And, of course, as I discussed in Chapter 5, do not forget to laugh at least 15 minutes every day!

Step 3:

Release to Relieve

"The best of perfections is immaculacy and the freeing of oneself from every defect. Once the individual is, in every respect, cleansed and purified, then will he become a focal center reflecting the Manifest Light."

'Abdu'l-Bahá

Once you are nourished, you have acquired the building blocks necessary to let go and to release, such as amino acids, vitamins, minerals, emotional support, and physical and inner strength. You are now ready for the third step in the KHOSH Method™: 'Release to Relieve'.

This step involves releasing what no longer serves you physically, physiologically, energetically, mentally, emotionally, socially and spiritually. In this step, it is important that you identify and clear the unnecessary baggage – the physical, emotional, mental, environmental and social toxins. Once you release, detox and depurate these toxins, you will gain a strong sense of relief, a stronger sense of self. It gives your body relief from the chronic physical and emotional pain resulting from carrying all that baggage. Your body will feel lighter, your energy more vibrant, your mind clearer, and your soul more elated. As you let go, you will find you stand up taller.

To eliminate the toxic load in your body and to create a youthful force within your being, you need to identify the imbalances, the root causes, and the initiators of imbalances within you. These may include your food intolerances and sensitivities, chemical toxins, infections and heavy metal exposure. In Appendix C you will find the root causes of aging and common toxins that interfere with your nervous system and promote inflammation and cellular aging. Identifying these suspects and learning to let go of them helps relieve the body, mind and spirit of the burdens that have been weighing down your system, creating inflammation, slowing cellular repair, causing hormonal imbalance, disrupting your microbiome, and promoting faster aging.

Releasing helps relieve your pains – both emotional and physical pain. It helps release the stress of the subconscious burdens you may be carrying from childhood events or generational old patterns and energies that are affecting your physical health, your mind and emotions. Removing the physical toxins allows you to access the deeper emotional and energetic burdens. The more you clear the emotional burdens, the healthier your cells.

Every time you experience a physical cleansing process, you may have an 'Aha' moment on an emotional or spiritual level. The purer your physical body becomes, the more you are able to elevate to higher spiritual frequencies. And the higher the spiritual state you access, the more your body is ready to let go of deeper cellular toxins. The deeper you access the cellular level and the more elevated you become spiritually, the more you reflect and receive 'Light', which further helps you propel through this world joyfully and more fulfilled, while achieving your purpose.

Detoxification and drainage for different substances varies during this step. For instance, heavy metal detox or chelation is different from a parasitic detox or a hormone detox. At this stage, you will need direction and guidance from your licensed naturopathic doctor to help you through the process. This third step may need to be periodically revisited as you move through the various steps of the KHOSH Method™ and gain the ability to access deeper layers of physical, mental, emotional and spiritual blockages.

Elimination Time

This step of 'release to relieve' starts with clean water, clean air and food therapy: following a diet of clean, organic and unprocessed whole plant-based foods. It involves continuing to eliminate food allergies and sensitivities while identifying your toxic load and infections.

Once these toxins have been identified, you can eliminate them through a systematic process using primary tools such as food therapy, IV nutrients, ozone therapy, natural antimicrobials, supplements and hydrotherapy, and secondary tools such as prescription medications. This step involves consulting your physician so they can diagnose the toxins and infections needing to be eliminated, and then oversee the detoxification process to reduce the risk of complications.

You may have already identified and reduced exposure to some things in step one, but this time you are going deeper to cleanse yourself of stubborn or persisting substances like molds, viruses, bacteria, parasites, and spirochetes and their toxins. Most importantly, in this step you are eliminating these one at a time as you dive into deeper cellular layers.

Once you have identified a root cause, you must let it go or eliminate it. As you eliminate each root cause, the ones hidden underneath it will surface and need to be eliminated too. This third step takes time. You may find yourself repeating this step a few times, and you may return to it after Step four as more layers are revealed that need to be released.

As you let go, you may experience 'Herx' (Herxheimer) reactions as your immune system wakes up to fight other layers[7], or as your body tries to figure out a path of elimination and drainage. You may be experiencing a Herx reaction when you feel flu-like symptoms of nausea, vomiting, fatigue, brain fog, body aches, chill, fever, headache and irritability. The use of binders, which are substances that bind toxins so to eliminate them through the bowels, can be helpful and necessary during this time. Optimizing your depuration systems (sweating, breathing, urinating, and bowel elimination) can also be helpful to minimize Herx reactions.

Be patient with yourself and the process. See Appendix D for tools you may use to help you release and let go.

Drainage for Healing

Optimizing drainage helps reduce Herx reactions, pain and toxic build-up. It helps relieve physical and emotional pain. When you clean your kitchen and are left with the dirty water in the sink, you have to pull the plug to drain the toxic water out of the sink. The same is true for our bodies. We must ensure drainage is activated to help the body drain its inflammatory cytokines and toxins.

As we learnt in Chapter 10, drainage is a safe and gentle process of normalizing the body's inflammation, elimination and detoxification processes using homeopathic remedies. Drainage impacts both internal and external cellular inflammation and elimination processes. It is not a quick fix; it works to assist the body's physiology to return to its normal processes. The idea is to reduce inflammation and create balance, healing and self-regulation.

Drainage focuses first on the primary organs of elimination, namely the liver, lungs, kidneys and intestines. When these primary organs are compromised, we often see symptoms in the secondary organs: the skin, mucous membranes, nose and genital organs. For example, the skin can break out in acne or eczema when the liver, lungs, intestines or kidneys are overly burdened. Improving their drainage helps reduce skin inflammation and improve the skin condition.

Drainage remedies include low-potency homeopathic remedies made from minerals, organs and plants. They work to activate normal cellular and organ physiology to eliminate toxins. Oligo elements are essential catalysts that act as enzymes to regulate cellular metabolism and support the body's terrain. Tissue salts or cell salts provide essential minerals that are needed for healthy cellular function. And, finally, we use gemmotherapies made from the sprouts or germination of plants. That first sprout often is filled with vital potent energy and concentrated nutrients that help support the plant into full growth. The energy and nutrients from plants help improve the body's drainage of toxins, cleanse metabolic wastes and support organ function. They also assist in emotional and energetic drainage.

I have seen many times how drainage, along with an anti-inflammatory diet, can produce extraordinary results. One such patient was a 78-year-old woman experiencing nausea, emotional stress, chronic tickborne infections, eczema, depression and anxiety, insomnia, chronic liver pain and debilitating fatigue. When she started the anti-inflammatory diet, she saw mild improvements.

We then introduced drainage remedies for liver, gallbladder, kidneys and lymphatic system.

Initially she was so weak we applied these topically, then when she became strong enough and started to improve, we introduced them orally. Her skin completely cleared. Her anxiety and depression resolved and her energy improved. Her sleep and appetite improved. She became stronger, more vibrant and happier. She was now ready for a deeper layer of detoxification and elimination of infections and toxins.

Sweat to Release

One of the easiest and most effective ways your body can release toxins is through the skin, through sweating. Heating the body and sweating, through sauna bathing, has been used as a natural depuration process in many cultures for centuries – and the benefits are now being confirmed by science. For instance, sweating by using a sauna supports immune function, reduces risks of acute and chronic illness, and lowers risks for pneumonia and heart disease[8]. The more often we take a sauna each week, the greater the benefits.

As part of this third step of the KHOSH Method™, make sure you are sauna bathing at least four times per week for 15 to 20 minutes. It is important to work up to higher temperatures slowly, and to acclimatize your system if you never have sauna bathed before. Start at a low temperature for a few minutes and then gradually increase the temperature and the time spent sauna bathing.

I prefer infrared sauna bathing as infrared rays penetrate deeper, burning toxins and fat surrounding inner organs like the liver and heart, and longer periods in the sauna can be tolerated better than in the traditional dry sauna. Make sure you stay hydrated as you sauna. After sauna bathing in the morning, taking a two- to five-minute cold shower activates your cellular mitochondria and improves cardiovascular health. In the evenings, you may prefer to use only a lukewarm rinse to help improve your sleep. Again, check with your physician to make sure sauna bathing is appropriate for your condition. You might want to check out shop.holistique.com for home care products like saunas that I recommend.

Fasting

Fasting, the act of intentionally abstaining from food for a period of time, is one of the main ways of physically and spiritually cleansing and detoxifying our body and soul. Fasting has been an integral part of human life for survival, health and wellbeing for centuries. Animals in the wild naturally fast periodically. Bears, for instance, fast in autumn and winter during hibernation. This ancient practice is regarded as a physical and a spiritual cleanse in many world faiths, cultures and traditions.

I like to think of fasting as one of the two most important pillars for sustaining health and stimulating the soul, the other being prayer. Medical fasting was first instigated in the 5th century by the Greek physician Hippocrates, the Father of Medicine, to treat certain conditions. Physiologically, fasting has been used to treat and prevent conditions of aging while also addressing overall health, longevity and prevention.

Fasting supports spiritual wellbeing, healthy blood sugar and insulin regulation as well as promotes healthy gut microbiome, enhanced mood and lipid metabolism[9]. As a result, fasting can reduce blood pressure and cholesterol and improve cardiovascular health. Fasting for longer than 16 days promotes weight loss while optimizing the release of neurochemicals. For instance, growth hormone increases during fasting as does serotonin, your natural antidepressant, and endorphins, your 'feel good' hormones[10].

It is important to include periods of refeeding following intermittent fasting to support cellular growth and structural remodeling. Remember, intermittent fasting is abstaining from food for 13 to 24 hours (usually for 13 to 17 hours) followed by a day of regular feeding. Intermittent fasting provides an easy way to reduce caloric intake to activate the cellular mitochondria to stay youthful, healthy and actively produce energy. Incidentally, calorie restriction through intermittent fasting or by following plant-based diets is one of the best ways to block all genes involved in aging while activating anti-aging genes. For the benefits of intermittent fasting, see GoldenGateBook.com/resources.

When To Fast or Cleanse

Fasting and cleansing is very different for women compared to men, whose hormones are relatively uniform with minor variations. Women ideally need to fast and cleanse according to their cycle to see optimum benefits and hormone regulation – especially in their premenopausal, or cycling, years. Dr. Mindy Pelz recommends the specifics of a fasting schedule for women in her book, *Fast Like a Girl*. For instance, abstain from fasting during the week leading up to your period, and reduce the hours of fasting to less than 17 hours during ovulation.

Most women crave carbs in the week prior to menses because progesterone production needs carbs, so eat them. Focus on healthy complex carbs like sweet potatoes, quinoa, millet, rice, and some fruit. During the first part of your cycle, your estrogen feeds off healthy fats and proteins, so enjoy a plant-based diet that is high in healthy fats – such as avocados, flaxseeds and pumpkin seeds – and low in carbs.

I have never seen a cycling woman do well on a long-term daily caloric-restriction fast, or on a long-term ketogenic diet (a high fat, low carb diet). Consistent long-term fasting without refeeding, or adopting a long-term ketogenic diet carried out in discord with your cycle, tends to elevate stress hormones[11] and reduce DHEA hormone[12].

This impacts thyroid function and activates your sympathetic nervous system, making you feel wired and tired[13]. Fasting can lead to urinary excretion of metals and cause hormonal imbalance, hair loss, irregular or missed cycles, mood changes, weight gain, and challenging perimenopausal symptoms especially if you are mineral deficient[14].

Your body needs periodic breaks from fasting to help reduce the stress/cortisol response. Hence, a pattern of intermittent fasting followed by one to three days of refeeding supports healthier hormone balance. One easy way to achieve ketosis is to follow intermittent fasting based on your cycle, rather than a long-term ketogenic diet. If you are menopausal or postmenopausal, fasting for 13 to 24 hours once to thrice a week can mitigate inflammation[15], reduce your waistline[16], improve insulin resistance[17] and improve your brain and heart health[18,19].

Intense detoxification or cleanse protocols, and intense exercise, should be avoided during the first three days of your menses as your body is already letting go and may weaken further with intense detoxification programs. However, you may be able to handle a modified fast or lower caloric intake as estrogen tends to suppress appetite. A miso or bone broth fast or higher intake of bone broth during those few days of your period can support your iron and mineral levels while healing the gut and supporting estrogen levels.

Foods to Support Liver Detoxification

As you have learned in previous chapters in Virtue II, detoxification is a biochemical process in the liver that helps eliminate toxins. Phase I liver detoxification is vital to maintaining healthy hormones, wellbeing and youthful aging. It is like emptying the fridge of leftovers and spoiled food. Phase I detoxification promotes the detoxification of drugs and medications and occurs through the cytochrome P450 enzymes in the liver. Phase II protects against oxidative damage and mutations of cells that could become cancerous.

Studies show certain foods support Phase I and Phase II detoxification. Certain teas, such as green tea, black tea and rooibos tea, protect against cancer thanks to their high polyphenol content[20]. Incorporating these foods into your daily diet supports regular detoxification pathways in your liver. See Appendix E for a list of foods, vitamins and amino acids that support Phase I and Phase II detoxification and glutathione.

Elimination of Infections

Many of us carry chronic infections like yeast, mold toxins (called mycotoxins), bacteria, spirochetes, parasites and/or viruses and their toxins, called biotoxins. Some of these infections may persist or become chronic like Long COVID-19, chronic mono (from Epstein-Barr virus), or chronic yeast infections. These chronic infections are often accompanied by disturbances in the gut microbiome (dysbiosis), inducing further inflammation which can set you up for chronic diseases. Part of this step of the KHOSH Method™ is to identify the imbalances or the presence of these infections and related toxins and reduce their load on the immune system, thereby freeing up the immune system to address more superficial insults like allergies while driving down chronic inflammation. It is not about sterilizing your system because sterilization creates disease as well. It is about bringing these microbes into balance within your system to promote your individualized healthy microbiome that will support a healthy immune function, optimize your hormones, calm your nervous system, improve mood and contribute to overall wellbeing.

Sometimes these infections are rooted in stealth infections in the mouth, gums, teeth or jawbone. A biological dentist should be able to identify any hidden infections in your mouth, around root canals, or in areas of dental extractions (known as cavitations) using 3-D cone X-ray and a live microscopic evaluation of your dental plaque.

This third step, in general, requires you to see a functional naturopathic physician who understands the implications and the chronicity of these infections, often hidden, and their impact on your health, symptoms and longevity. The physician should perform a comprehensive evaluation and testing for infections, and an assessment of your microbiome, to understand the infectious load and their insult on your health. A list of lab tests that may be used to diagnose the infectious load in your body and your immune status can be found at **GoldenGateBook.com/resources**.

Chronic infections should ideally be treated with biological non-invasive therapies first. Many of the anti-microbial herbal medicines, for instance berberine, not only fight infections but also modulate the microbiome, act as an anti-inflammatory and support healthy immune function[21]. In this step, I may also incorporate ozone therapy, therapeutic peptides, IV Vitamin C, hyperbaric oxygen therapy[22], Specific Oligonucleotide Therapy (SOT) and much more when treating chronic and acute infections and immune function[23].

Ozone therapy, for instance, can potentially inactivate infections – especially viruses, including SARS-CoV-2[25], herpes simplex, influenza A and Ebola. Ozone therapy can also inhibit even antibiotic-resistant bacteria[26,27]. Intravenous Vitamin C (ascorbic acid) therapy is showing promise in the treatment of acute and chronic infections, including Sars-CoV-2, and bacterial sepsis[28]. Hyperbaric oxygen therapy acts as a potent antimicrobial[29] and has been shown to effectively treat viruses, including Long COVID-19[30].

Antisense therapy, or SOT, is a novel targeted gene therapy approach that uses protein chains (oligonucleotides) specific to the individual's infection. The specific oligonucleotide binds to the mRNA of the specific infection and slows the replication of the infection. SOT can currently be created for certain bacterial, viral, and spirochete infections[31,32].

Elimination of Chronic Heavy Metal Toxicity

As part of this third step of the KHOSH Method™, chronic heavy metal toxicity plays a big role in chronic and aging diseases, chronic infections and hormonal imbalances[33]. Chronic heavy metal toxicity contributes to cardiovascular disease, which presents a far greater risk of mortality for women than men, and infertility[34]. It also induces breast cancer and other age-related diseases[35,36]. It induces oxidative stress and impedes proteins and enzymes[37]. It is therefore vital to identify and release heavy metals to reverse aging and inflammation – especially in the blood vessels and the heart.

Heavy metal toxicity differs from heavy metal poisoning because heavy metal poisoning is an emergency requiring acute hospital care, while toxicity is a slow accumulation of metals that may go unnoticed for years. Chronic ambiguous symptoms like neuropathy, numbness and tingling, acne, hair loss, hormonal issues, a silver hue around the eyes, digestive symptoms, heart issues and fatigue are examples of symptoms of people with chronic heavy metal toxicity.

Metal toxicity promotes aging of cells and inflammation by influencing gene expression[38], accelerating senescence[39], shortening telomeres, blocking DNA transcription and vitamin D synthesis[40] and weakening cell membranes. Metals act as hormone disruptors[41] that increase the risks for cancers, infertility and hormone imbalance, and worsen perimenopausal or postmenopausal symptoms. Metal toxicity is involved in osteoarthritis[42], Alzheimer's, brain inflammation and heart disease, and linked to chronic disease and aging[43]. For example, mercury found in tuna, swordfish and halibut is linked to autoimmune disease, thyroiditis and breast cancer. For a more comprehensive list of metal related symptoms and illnesses, refer to GoldenGateBook.com/resources.

The good news is that the majority of the effects of heavy metal toxicity can be reversed by removing metals from the body through chelation[44] – a process of binding metals to help the body eliminate them. Chelation allows your hormone glands to rebalance their hormone production and function, and lets your immune system gain more vitality. When the metal load in your body is reduced, DNA transcription and vitamin D synthesis begin to re-establish, senescence slows, telomere lengthening improves, and the integrity of cellular membranes is enhanced.

A recent study shows the importance of the chelation of metals in treating heart disease, diabetes and atherosclerosis[45]. Nerve toxicity caused by lead, for example, can be reversed with cilantro[46]. Chelation should be done under the supervision of a licensed physician who understands the complexity and risks of heavy metal detoxification. For a list of agents used in the chelation of metals, and nutrients that support chelation, please see **GoldenGateBook.com/resources**.

Methods of testing for heavy metal toxicity include analysis of blood, urine or hair, and spectrophotometry, which detects intracellular levels of heavy metals by beaming full spectrum light onto the palm of your hand and measuring the intensity of the light absorbed[47]. I prefer using spectrophotometry because it is non-invasive and quick and sensitive to detecting intracellular metal accumulation[48]. While blood levels detect acute toxicity, hair analysis detects the readily released metals and not the ones that are tightly bound inside the cells of the body, like mercury. Urine tests check the body's capacity to eliminate metals through the kidneys but do not identify the intracellular metals that are stuck within the cells.

Chemical Upset

The plethora of chemicals we breathe, touch, eat, smell, drink or are injected with bombard our entire system. They cause inflammation, cellular dysfunction, genetic mutations and hormone disruptions, making us sicker and older faster while increasing our cancer risks. Toxic chemicals potentially affect every organ function, alter mood and hormone regulation, and cause detoxification problems, cellular death, and even changes in the mitochondria and the nervous system[49].

Glyphosate, for example, the most commonly used pesticide that is the active ingredient in Roundup, can be inhaled, consumed or touched. Exposures to glyphosate through air, food, occupational exposure and touch have been shown to activate oxidative stress, cause organ and mitochondrial damage, induce inflammation and pro-inflammatory cytokines, lead to nervous system toxicity, and cause DNA damage – all of which promote cancer growth, infertility, miscarriage, gene expression disruptions, nervous system disorders and intestinal diseases, as well as liver, kidney, and lung conditions in humans and animals[50,51].

It is like pouring bleach on your favorite blue sweater. Before your eyes, you see the blue disappear. If you leave the bleach long enough, you will see holes in your sweater as the bleach burns through. The same kind of reaction happens in our bodies when we consume foods containing pesticides, herbicides or chemical preservatives, or we drink sugar-free soda containing aspartame and artificial sweeteners. Our cells are getting burnt and holes are being created in our bodily functions, contributing to the hallmarks of aging.

Identifying the chemical load accumulated over the years, and then detoxifying and depurating them, can help counteract some of the damage that such chemicals cause. Incorporating bitter melon in your diet for example[52], along with vitamin C, curcumin[53] and zinc supplementation[54] have been shown to protect against chemical toxicity. Furthermore, think about some of the techniques previously discussed in this book, such as sauna bathing, IV glutathione therapy and diet and lifestyle modifications, as important tools to detoxify chemicals in this third step of the KHOSH Method™.

Bind It and Let It Go!

As you release infections, heavy metals, chemicals and toxins from your tissues and lymphatic system, it is vital to make sure they are eliminated through the bowels and urine. Binding agents such as zeolite, fulvic acid, chlorella, calcium d-glucarate, activated charcoal, silica, apple pectin, humic acid and modified citrus pectin can act as effective binders to help remove hormone metabolites, toxins or infections. This binding step is vital to reduce the reabsorption of toxins through the colon wall back into the blood system, known as enterohepatic recirculation.

A vital part of this third step is the emotional release that frequently accompanies the physical release, or it may be done on its own. The emotional stressors, conflicts, trauma and harbored emotions we carry can block the release of the physical toxins. They act as magnets to keep parasites, other infections, chemicals or metal toxins in place, for instance.

As you let go of the physical parasite, you also need to let go of any interferences in your emotional, energetic and spiritual relationship with your host. A dysfunctional relationship with your mother, for instance, your very first physical and emotional host, can continue to attract physical parasites. Resolving any dysfunction you hold in your cells relating to this maternal relationship will ensure the complete release of physical parasites and reduce the risk of them re-attaching to you.

A 48 year old perimenopausal woman complaining of nausea, abdominal pain and constipation along with insomnia, anxiety and hot flashes came to see me. We identified parasitic infections and assumed it was in the gallbladder since her gallbladder was tender on examination. Using multiple herbal combinations, homeopathic drainage remedies, binders, and Ondamed therapy, we treated the parasites. Her symptoms resolved temporarily until we cleared her of the emotional resentment she carried of her mother leaving her when she was a child. She then learnt to replace her resentment with gratitude and compassion for her mother for teaching her resilience and independence. Her symptoms resolved and never returned again.

Your Order is Unique

Step three of the KHOSH Method™ can be complicated. The order in which toxins, infections, chemicals and hormones are released and eliminated is highly individualized. It is like cutting through a layered cake. In order to get to the bottom of the cake, one must cut through each layer. Compounded in each layer are the multitude layers of emotional and ancestral traumas, physical toxins and energetic baggage we carry. The stacking of layers is different for each person and often requires an objective specialist to understand each of the layers and identify the order of their removal for your particular body.

For your health to improve and to help you age gracefully, the order and timing of removing and eliminating these toxins makes all the difference between a successful therapeutic approach and one that is not so effective. That is the art of medicine, which I feel is the most unique reason why you would pick one physician over another to help you with your personal journey.

Step three requires you to trust the process and believe that it will lead you to wellbeing and joy so you can fulfill your destiny and purpose.

Step 4:

Restore to Heal

"The soul always knows
what to do to heal itself.
The challenge
is to silence the mind."

Caroline Myss

Now that you have reduced, replenished, nourished, released and removed toxins, it is time to restore your cells and tissues. Your cells are now hungry for more nourishment – for healing. Your cells know what they need to restore themselves. You just need to stop interfering. Instead provide space, time, patience, and resources for your body's healing. Silence your mind. Silence your need to do something. Practice to just 'be'. Be patient. Be kind. Be love to your cells.

In this step, similar to the replenishment step, your cells need nourishment with oxygen, vitamins, minerals, amino acids, fatty acids and hormones. Breathe, drink lots of clean filtered water (I recommend half your body weight in ounces), get fresh air, eat organic whole foods, take exercise and sleep. Sleep is the best way to restore your body because during sleep the body secretes the highest amount of growth hormone, which activates the healing and restoration of cells. Sleep can also profoundly restore mental, emotional and body functions, especially after a stressful event[55].

When cells are cleaned out, fuel needs to be put in. Think about what happens when you re-pot a plant. First, you trim its dead leaves and remove unhealthy soil. Then you place your plant into a pot and fill the pot with fresh, healthy nutrient-rich soil along with water, sunlight and fresh air. This helps the plant grow faster and more vibrantly.

We need to do the same with our bodies. Once we have cleaned it out, we need to replace the nutrients, oxygen, water, minerals and so forth. When metals are removed from cells, mineral deficiency becomes strongly evident, and it becomes vital to replenish them to restore cellular function. When the body's load of bacteria, viruses, parasites and yeast is reduced, beneficial bacteria need to be replaced to restore the microbiome and activate a healthy digestive function.

Nutrient testing to identify nutritional deficiencies becomes useful at this stage. This can identify the nutrients you are low on – for instance, Vitamin D, K2 or A, which all play an important role in establishing a healthy gut, mucous membranes, mitochondria and immune functions[56]. Biotin and essential omega-3 fatty acids, such as fish oil and flaxseeds, help restore the gut microbiome and its diversity without the need for probiotics supplementation[57]. Methylated B-vitamins, zinc, magnesium and n-acetyl cysteine may be needed to support your ongoing detoxification system.

During this fourth stage, I restore healing and repair the gut, its microbiome, bones and skin by using bone broth, warming stews, herbal teas[58] and plant oils – such as coconut oil[59], olive oil[60], rose oil[61] and avocado oil[62]. When estrogen levels decline during menopause, and the skin becomes dry and wrinkled, a topical application of virgin coconut oil[63], ozonated olive oil[64] and rosehip oil[65] can be restorative. Regular intake of flaxseeds can be corrective during menopause, reducing menopausal symptoms and supporting estrogen metabolism[66].

I support my estrogen levels by adding 1 to 2 tablespoons of freshly ground organic flaxseeds and hemp seeds to 100% grassfed Greek yogurt or a chia pudding most mornings. Regular tea-drinking, make sure it's organic, can protect against menopause-related memory decline because of its polyphenols content[67]. Different species of maca, a plant known for its adaptogenic properties, can help restore hormone balance during premenopause, perimenopause, menopause, and premenopause[68].

Drainage and Homeopathic Remedies

One of my favorite ways to restore, repair and heal tissues, cellular function and hormones is through the use of drainage remedies such as Pleo Sanum, Gemmotherapy, Pekana, Desbio remedies and other bioregulatory medicines. These remedies are rooted in the European homeopathic medical system, dating back more than 300 years.

Gemmotherapies use phytonutrients from young shoots/buds of plants to regulate cellular metabolism and function[69]. Pekana, Desbio, Pleo Sanum and Heel remedies use low potency combination homeopathic medicines, which regulate and bring into homeostasis the various functions within the body: our physiological, mental, emotional, nutritional, structural, and bioenergetic systems while activating cellular vitality[70].

Fasting

In addition to being an important tool in Step Three, Release to Relieve, fasting can also be used to restore the gut, its microbiome and the circadian rhythm in Step Four[71]. For instance, a seven-day water fast under medical supervision appears to be restorative to the gut microbiome[72]. And intermittent fasting (alternating days of 13 to 17-hour fast from the last meal the night before), combined with dietary fiber, appears to be restorative to the gut microbiome, immune function and weight management[73].

A 48-hour fast improves insulin sensitivity and activates cellular repair. A 19-day dry fast - no eating or drinking from dawn to dusk - enhances mindfulness and wellbeing, while improving cholesterol, blood sugar, inflammation, energy and stress tolerance.

Prebiotics and Probiotics

Foods promoting the growth of your personal signature of beneficial bacteria are important to include at this stage. Green bananas, kudzu, cooled cooked rice and potatoes are good examples of resistant starch which promote a healthy gut microbiome and potentially improve blood sugar regulation and insulin resistance[74].

They are all considered prebiotics. Green banana flour, for example, has been shown to quickly restore the gut microbiome even after the gut microbiome becomes disrupted with antibiotic therapy[75]. Fermented foods like Greek yogurt and kefir, or fermented vegetables like sauerkraut help improve the microbiome and blood-sugar control even in diabetics[76].

Probiotics have historically been used to replace gut bacteria. While they were once promoted as an important health supplement, they are not always useful for everyone during this stage of restoration. In patients with high-risk conditions – for instance those with immune deficiency cancer, sepsis, pneumonia, or heart infections – probiotics may worsen conditions by causing infections. In patients with leaky gut, diabetes, certain malignancies, and post-organ transplant issues, probiotic supplementation does not seem to make a difference[77]. On the other hand, probiotic Bifidobacterium supplementation can improve memory and mild cognitive decline[78].

Using lifestyle and food therapy[79], yoga[80], homeopathy, restorative meditation[81], breathing exercises and stress management techniques to restore the gut microbiome can often be more powerful and safer than using over-the-counter store-bought probiotic[82] supplementation. If you are experiencing chronic health concerns or hormonal imbalance,

I recommend you reach out to my clinic, Holistique.com, to see one of our licensed naturopathic physicians who can properly assess your gut microbiome and correct it using diet, nutrition, prebiotics and appropriate probiotics if necessary.

Peptide Therapy

Peptide therapy can be a useful tool during this restorative fourth step as well as the next regenerative step of the KHOSH Method™. Peptides, like insulin, are short chains of amino acids that act as signaling molecules or communication systems in the body, and may also act as restorative agents. There are over 4,000 peptides in the body but only a few are used therapeutically for now. Peptides may be taken as topical treatments, orally, as a nasal spray, or as injectable therapy. The FDA is currently attempting to regulate the compounding and prescription of some of these peptides. Therefore, not all therapeutic peptides are available in the USA, but they may be found in Europe and Australia.

Examples of therapeutic peptides and their medical uses include the antiaging peptide Epithalamin. It is produced by the pineal gland which restores immune activity, the antioxidant system, and reproductive function[83]. MOTS-c, a mitochondrial-derived peptide, signals the repair of mitochondria function[84]. Applying Zinc-thymulin and GHK-Cu peptides topically helps restore hair, skin and youthful beauty. Thymosin beta-4 galvanizes immune function, and Semax helps re-establish neurocognitive function, reducing the risk of brain damage in Alzheimer's sufferers[85].

Other peptides include KPV[86], which helps repair the gut[87] and the microbiome, and SS-31[88], which has antiaging benefits and restores mitochondrial function. DSIP[89] restores circadian rhythm to improve sleep, Cerebrolysin[90] heals brain neurons and function, and the BPC-157[91] peptide repairs muscles, tendons, gut lining and the gut-brain axis.

A 78-year-old gentleman with Parkinson's disease came to my clinic presenting with tremors, anxiety, instability walking, and fatigue. I started treating him with oral BPC-157, Semax and KPV nasal sprays, and Cerebrolysin therapy. Within a month, his walking became significantly more stable, his tremors improved, his anxiety declined, his energy progressed and he regained a general sense of wellbeing and joy.

Ozone and Hyperbaric Oxygen Therapies

As you learned in Step Three of the KHOSH Method™, ozone therapy (O3) provides oxygen to cells, so cells can use O3 to restore and repair tissue. In some countries, ozone therapy is used as an antiaging therapy[92] for both the skin and internal systems like the cardiovascular[93], metabolic[94], nervous and hormonal systems[95].

Ozone supports healing of the mitochondria and enhances the cells' antioxidant system to reduce oxidative stress. This reduces inflammation, blood pressure and arterial inflammation while regulating blood sugar and brain function. Hence, ozone therapy acts as a potent antiaging therapy[96,97]. Ozone therapy may also reduce pain, especially in fibromyalgia and musculoskeletal conditions, and stimulate healing of both osteoarthritis and rheumatoid arthritis[98].

Hyperbaric oxygen therapy (HBOT) repairs the tissues of the gut, brain[100], heart, skin, nervous system[101], muscle, bones and cartilage. It increases telomere length[102] and also stimulates homeostasis in the body[103]. Because HBOT improves cell-to-cell communication, mitigates inflammation, improves stress response, modulates immune function and activates repair processes in the body, it acts as a fantastic restoration therapy[104].

Injection Therapies

Intravenous (IV) nutrient therapies are very useful during this restorative step of the KHOSH Method™ to provide nutrition directly to the cells. Bypassing the gut and administering higher dose of nutrients intravenously boosts the restoration of cells, immunity, the nervous system, skin and hormones. Nutrients commonly administered intravenously to meet the cells' nutritional demand during healing are B-vitamins, magnesium, zinc, potassium, calcium, vitamin C, minerals and amino acids. I also use IV hydration, containing minerals, to provide the hydration and mineral levels cells need to revive their cellular function and health.

Bio-Identical Hormone Therapy

During this restorative stage, bio-identical hormone therapies (BHRT) may be prescribed to support your body's cellular restoration and function. Hormone balance is an integral and crucial component of a healthy mind, body and spirit. You may need to look back to Chapters 13 and 14 to review the importance of BHRT for health and vitality.

Therapies using bio-identical testosterone, estriol (E3), estradiol (E2), progesterone, DHEA (a hormone produced by the adrenal gland), oxytocin and pregnenolone revitalize mitochondrial and cellular health when these hormones are either insufficiently produced or in too great demand. BHRT may be prescribed to perimenopausal,

menopausal or postmenopausall women after comprehensive blood, saliva and urine testing. I find the DUTCH hormone panel to be the most comprehensive, especially when combined with blood levels of hormones. Bio-identical hormone therapy may be compounded in a variety of forms and dosages: creams, suppositories, oral drops, capsules or pellets. Not all these forms are recommended or available for all hormones. For instance, testosterone should never be taken orally. It can be applied vaginally, topically or in pellet form. Estradiol (E2) is available as a patch, topical or vaginal cream, suppository, pellet and sublingual drops. But E2 should never be taken orally, because it can be processed by the liver into more toxic metabolites.

Other Restorative Tools to Use

Light therapy can be used topically, as either a low-level laser or red-light therapy, for wound healing and skin and hair rejuvenation. It can also be used intravenously, as photodynamic laser light therapy combined with photosensitizing agents, to fight cancer[104], inflammation, and infections[105].

Low-level laser light therapy (LLLT) can be effective in restoring mitochondrial function, reducing inflammation and pain, and activating stem-cell function to heal injuries[106] and wounds, rejuvenate skin[107], and fight infections, cancer and autoimmune conditions[108].

Emotional and Spiritual Restoration

In Step Three of the KHOSH Method™, you released the emotional, mental and energetic baggage you may have carried for years. In this restorative step, it is time to restore your emotional, mental and energetic wellbeing by nurturing yourself with time – time to be, to reflect, to see, and to connect.

During this step, you will want to focus on practicing positive virtues, such as loving and forgiving yourself, being patient and grateful, and providing the space for your healing and restoration. You may need to make time to meditate, to pray, to reflect, to go for a walk, to sing, to dance, to consult with others, to let things be, or just learn to have faith that all will be okay. You may need to learn to trust. Trust the Universe. Trust the process. Trust your body's capacity to heal. Trust you have been endowed with the innate tools within your body to regenerate itself.

In this step, prayer, meditation and reflection become essential to heal the body, mind and soul. Once you have prayed, sit quietly and reflect. I find it helpful to reflect every night and bring myself to account before I sleep. You may want to jot down your thoughts and feelings in a journal every night before bed. There is no room for self-criticism – there is only room for love and patience. Focus on visualizing the love and light that is coming into the crown of your head from above. Feel the warmth, the nourishment, the restoration. You have the capacity to heal. Your body has the capacity to heal and restore. Allow yourself. Accept the love and light.

Now you have been replenished, released and restored, you are now ready for the next step in the KHOSH Method™: Regenerate to Create.

Step 5:

Regenerate to Create

"A new day, a new night;
new gardens, new life,
every breath brings
about fresh insights;
newness is richness,
joyfulness."

Rumi

With every day, with every breath, you have the opportunity to create a new version of yourself: one that fulfills your inner yearnings and brings you utmost inner joy. Now that you have reduced inflammation, replenished yourself with physical, emotional and spiritual food, released your toxins, infections, and associated emotions, and restored your hormones, nutrition, oxygen and spiritual connections, your system is prepared to regenerate to create a new you.

Regenerative medicine is an emerging medical specialty that aims to replenish, restore and regenerate cells, tissues, and organs to re-establish healthy human function. Scientists believe that regenerating your DNA and stem cells is the key to holding back aging and promoting longevity[109,110]. The process involves activating cells, especially the mitochondria, to help the body renew and repair itself.

We all age at different rates depending on factors such as our environmental exposures, nutrition, activity level, emotional stressors, microbiome and genetics. Women age fastest between the ages of 35 and menopause due to the decline in estrogen that wreaks havoc by damaging DNA and stem cells, and by increasing reactive oxygen species.

The goal to regenerate, therefore, is to address the Hallmarks of Aging as noted in Chapter 15: preserve DNA from damage while accelerating repair and regenerative mechanisms, sustaining estrogen levels, reducing inflammation, preserving or regenerating our stem cells, maintaining telomere length, correcting dysbiosis and slowing cell senescence.

Luckily, as research in aging and regenerative medicine continues, we have gained many tools to support the body's regenerative processes. The fifth step of the KHOSH Method™ focuses on these regenerative techniques and therapies that you may use under the guidance of a knowledgeable and licensed physician. These therapies will activate regenerative processes within your stem cells and DNA to improve telomere length and mitochondria function, slow senescence and mute (or perhaps even reverse) some of the aging processes.

Begin with centering yourself through breathing exercises, meditation and prayer – which often moves us into a meditative state. If you find it difficult to meditate, try using one of the multiple meditation apps available, or go to a yoga class. Meditation activates our immune system, reducing inflammation and improving brain energy[111]. Even after a short meditation, telomere lengths of DNA are lengthened[112], the stress response of our brain and nervous system is improved and hormones become more balanced[113].

Another recent study evaluating mind-body interventions like meditation and yoga found that the risk of heart disease in women significantly reduces as the structure and function of the brain changes, cortisol secretions balance, blood pressure and heart rate variability improve, and immune reactions modulate[114]. This all contributes to alleviating menopausal symptoms and positively impacting women's cardiovascular health.

I find that yoga can be a great starting point to shift your mind and thoughts towards wellbeing. It can induce stem cell trafficking, which is when stem cells migrate to new areas of the body to activate tissue repair and regeneration, thereby slowing aging[115]. Stem cell trafficking supports a healthier liver function, delays skin wrinkles, enhances heart function and insulin regulation, reduces belly fat, improves memory and focus, and increases lung capacity.

Once you start meditation, then add in a plant-based diet, sleep, relaxation and breathing techniques, intermittent fasting, and regular exercise – all the things we have discussed in the previous steps of the KHOSH Method™. Starting a plant-based, whole foods diet and healthy lifestyle practices such as hydrotherapy, sauna therapy and intermittent fasting are the cornerstones of regenerative medicine. Do not forget to incorporate spices and herbs like turmeric, cumin, saffron, garlic, rosemary, basil, oregano and thyme to further activate your cells' regenerative processes and reduce inflammation.

I find that in many cases, especially if you are in perimenopause or menopausal, bioidentical hormone therapy, plus peptide and oxygen therapies, can also boost your cellular regenerative processes in this stage. Let's explore more regenerative tools that are at your disposal at our comprehensive regenerative clinic **Holistique.com**, in Bellevue, Washington.

Ozone and Oxygen Therapies

Ozone and oxygen therapies, which are useful tools in the first four steps of the KHOSH Method™, can also be effective in this regenerative stage. The hallmark of aging is mitochondria dysfunction, and ozone therapies promote the regeneration of the mitochondria[116] including in COVID-19 cases[117] and in peripheral vascular disease[118]. If the mitochondria can be regenerated and supported, and the antioxidant system is activated, then cellular energy increases and aging potentially slows. Low-dose ozone therapy can activate the antioxidant system in the mitochondria[119], while high-dose ozone therapy can heal and regenerate the mitochondria[120].

Hyperbaric oxygen therapy (HBOT) improves mitochondrial dysfunction, optimizing its activity and regeneration to renew brain cells, skin, joints and heart cells[121]. After a few days of HBOT therapy, the skin looks more vibrant and youthfully free of blemishes. Joint pain and joint inflammation resolve and a general sense of wellbeing and uplifting energy generates.

NanoVi Therapy

Mitochondria dysfunction and damage sets in after the age of 25, when cellular aging begins and energy starts to decline. If you wish to unleash your feminine powers, the need for cellular regeneration heightens after this point. The NanoVi device promotes cellular regeneration by improving oxygen metabolism, optimizing the antioxidant defense mechanisms protecting cells against free radical damage, increasing cellular energy production, and correcting DNA protein folding. Regular use of NanoVi therapy enhances vitality, builds stronger immunity, increases oxygen uptake by cells, and optimizes cellular regeneration[122]. You may purchase a NanoVi device for home use from **shop.holistique.com**.

NanoVi therapy works by encouraging the initiation and restoration of protein folding, through bio-regulatory signaling of water molecules. To reap the benefits, simply breathe in the water molecule signals produced by the NanoVi device during a daily 20 to 30-minute session. Your brain often feels clear and energy improves shortly after. Ideally, use NanoVi therapy after an ozone or hyperbaric session to optimize the regeneration and antioxidant systems of the mitochondria.

Homeopathic Remedies

Homeopathic remedies, discovered in Germany in 1810 by Dr. Samuel Hahnemann, are dilutions of natural substances like minerals or plants that activate healing in cells and tissues. The effects of homeopathy have been denied in Western medicine, even though thousands of anecdotal reports from around the world and several recently published scientific studies have demonstrated its efficacy. The concept of vaccinations, incidentally, was originally based on the principles of homeopathy, which was initially called 'vaccinia'.

Even though homeopathy has been prescribed for over 200 years with positive outcomes, scientific research proving and understanding its effects and benefits are only recently underway. Research studies evaluating the efficacy of homeopathy and its role in medicine and in regeneration of tissues has been promising[123]. For instance, a study on rats using a homeopathic Hypericum perforatum 30c remedy, given orally twice a day for a week, successfully showed regeneration and recovery of the rats' peripheral nerve[124].

Another 2019 study showed that a homeopathy preparation of Symphytum officinalis activated regeneration of mesenchymal stem cells in bone marrow, suggesting that homeopathic Symphytum officinalis promotes osteogenesis (bone regeneration)[125]. Another in vivo study looking at the regeneration of skeletal muscle after injection of homeopathic medicines showed a faster regeneration of the muscle fiber by enhancing the 'pro-regenerative' genes in the muscle[126].

In another 2023 randomized, controlled, single-blind study of 129 COVID-19 patients, the addition of homeopathic remedies of Bryonia alba, Phosphorus, Arsenicum album, Tuberculinum bovinum, and

Arnica montana significantly reduced mortality and morbidity and laboratory markers[127].

I frequently prescribe homeopathic Arnica montana to repair tissues after surgery or trauma. A 2016 study provides an insight into Arnica's ability to modify and regulate key genes involved with tissue regeneration and repair, tissue remodeling and inflammation[128]. I prescribe homeopathy remedies not only because they work, but because they are safe, easy to take and effective. My experience shows that these powerful, yet subtle, remedies work if the correct remedy is prescribed at the correct dosage.

I raised my three daughters on homeopathic remedies. Instead of using anti-inflammatories and pain medications for injuries, teething and earaches, or antibiotics for infections, my girls received homeopathic remedies since their infancy. And when I had a second-degree tear in my calf muscle eight years ago, and was told that a full recovery would take months, I took matters into my own hands and began injecting homeopathic remedies into my calf muscle every other day. I was back on my feet within a week. And within two weeks, I had fully recovered and was able to run. As the science of medicine matures, I look forward to more scientific studies proving the known benefits of homeopathy, especially in regenerative medicine.

Prolotherapy, Prolozone, and Platelet Rich Plasma (PRP) Therapy

After the birth of my children, I began suffering from sciatic pain and lower back pain. An X-ray showed I had an extra lumbar vertebra: instead of five, I had six, making my pelvic unstable, especially after the trauma of childbirth. I began seeking out non-invasive therapies that would stabilize my sacroiliac joint and the lower lumbar joints by regenerating healing ligaments, tendons, discs and muscles.

I found prolotherapy, which is a technique that injects an irritant solution, like lidocaine and dextrose, into affected areas like tendons and ligaments to stimulate their regeneration and healing. While I was being trained in this technique, I received a single injection which resolved my pain and stabilized my lower back and pelvis. I was amazed.

A year later, I learnt about prolozone therapy. Ozone gas is injected into the injured or the degenerative joint and surrounding tissues. Because it is a gas, it spreads to the areas in the joint, tissues or the skin that need to heal. Since ozone is an analgesic (a pain reliever), prolozone therapy reduces pain as well as activates collagen and joint and skin repair[129,130]. It promotes skin and wound healing, hence it works wonders with skin discoloration, acne, and fine lines.

It was 2006 when I first heard about Platelet-Rich Plasma (PRP) therapy at a prolotherapy injection training seminar in Vancouver, Canada. I thought it was incredibly creative (and bizarre) to have your own blood plasma with its high concentration of platelets, seven growth factors and stem cells extracted and then reinjected into joints, tendons, ligaments and muscles to accelerate their healing, repair and regeneration. I was awed.

The use of PRP dates back to the 1970s when hematologists used it for blood clotting and healing. Later, in the 1980s, dental surgeons used it to clot and regenerate gums after dental surgery[131]. Injecting PRP into a joint, ligament, tendon, or skin creates a scab – similar to a scab you get after a cut on your skin.

It acts as an alarm that summons the body's immune and inflammatory responses to the injected site to repair, heal and regenerate it. For the first three to five days, while the scab promotes the active regeneration and healing mechanisms, it is recommended to avoid strenuous physical activities and any anti-inflammatory medications, so the body continues to use its own inflammatory process as a source of healing.

Soon after, in 2007, I realized that combining PRP and ozone therapy would be more effective for regenerating joints, skin, tissues, and collagen than either individually. I began using PRP with ozone to heal sports injuries, strains and sprains, arthritic and painful joints, and areas of pain along the spine. I also used it to rejuvenate facial skin, as a non-invasive gentle face and breasts lift, and for pelvic/vaginal rejuvenation and healing.

Fifteen years later, studies are now being published proving what I had discovered then: that there is less pain, faster healing and lower risk of infection when PRP is combined with ozone[132]. I began to see chronic knee, back and shoulder pain resolve, and joint mobility improve. PRP with ozone seems to be a miracle non-invasive therapy for these chronic degenerative and physical injuries. That was 2006. No one in Washington State was doing these injections at that time, and I was thrilled to bring these techniques to this area.

Five years later, I received a text from a friend about a new medical use of PRP, and thought that perhaps it would help hair grow. I was on the plane the next month, heading to Mobile, Alabama to train with Dr. Runnels, an emergency room doctor who had discovered new uses for PRP. He had discovered its benefits for hair growth, skin rejuvenation and remodeling facial muscles to create a gentle yet youthful face. It also improves sexual function and health when injected in the external reproductive systems of women and men.

Because PRP activates collagen regeneration, injecting it into the facial muscle, or micro-needling it into the face and neck, or even injecting it into the breast and vaginal tissues, stimulates tightening and lifting of skin and muscle. Within three weeks of the injection, you start to notice baby hairs growing after an injection into the scalp. Gradually, the lips naturally look a little fuller, the face is tighter and more youthful, the breasts are lifted and slightly fuller. Vaginal tissue feels more lubricated and healthier, orgasm is easier and pelvic pain has decreased.

PRP continues to regenerate tissues for months afterwards. Most patients see the full effects of PRP between four to six months after the first injections – providing they stick to the KHOSH Diet™ for at least a week prior to PRP collection. Access **GoldenGateBook.com/resources** to learn more about the KHOSH Longevity Diet™ I use to optimize PRP and regenerative injection therapies.

Stem Cell Therapy

The term 'stem cells' was coined in 1908 by Russian-American scientist Maximov. But it was not until 1960 that scientists published the first evidence of nerve regeneration in brain stem cells[133]. This marked the beginning of a new field of regenerative medicine focusing on repairing, renewing and regenerating cells, tissues and organs to re-establish function and health. Baby stem cells, instilled with so much vital force and regenerative power, are native cells with the ability to renew and regenerate themselves. Because they are not specialized cells with a specific function in the body, they can turn into a specialized cell like a muscle, bone, brain or blood cell.

Mesenchymal stem cells (MSCs) originate in the human embryo and are full of vitality and potentiality. MSCs can be found in bone-marrow, umbilical cord blood and tissue, fat, liver, amniotic fluid and other tissues. They self-renew and self-regenerate. They are multipotent, meaning they can become different tissues such as bone, nerve, fat, cartilage or liver cells. Umbilical cord MSCs have fast renewal capacity and have been shown to accumulate in inflamed or damaged tissue to promote tissue repair. They modulate immune system function, reduce inflammation and release cytokines to modulate the cell environment[134,135].

Today, MSCs are extracted either from bone marrow, fat tissue, umbilical cord blood and tissue (Wharton's jelly), or the placenta. These MSCs are used therapeutically to activate regeneration of skin, joints, collagen, tendons, brain neurons and heart cells[136], for instance. Bone-derived MSCs decline in number and quality with age – the older you get, the lower the number of stem cells, especially from your bone marrow[137,138]. Therefore, using bone marrow stem cells in someone who is in late perimenopause or postmenopause will not yield a high amount of viable stem cells to support repair and regeneration[139,140].

The most concentrated native MSCs are derived from Wharton's jelly (from umbilical cord tissue)[141]. Umbilical MSCs can be harvested non-invasively and easily. They modulate immune response, decrease inflammation and do not cause graft-host disease.

These baby cells promote tissue regeneration, reduce clotting and improve cellular environment[142]. MSCs may be used to treat infections, like COVID-19[143] and other bacterial infections[144]. Most of the scientific studies focusing on stem cell therapy for chronic disease such as Alzheimer's, Parkinson's, ALS, heart disease, autoimmune disease, including Type 1 Diabetes, and rheumatoid arthritis also use MSCs[145,146]. They can be used to support collagen and tissue regeneration along with ozone, PRP and peptide therapy.

Light Therapy

Light therapy is one of the most effective non-invasive regenerative therapies. Light made up of different wavelengths, applied topically, intravenously or vaginally, has multiple healing effects[147]. Each wavelength of light (red, yellow, green, blue, infrared and ultraviolet light), its duration and dose of exposure supports the body's natural regenerative processes, hormone and immune functions in different ways to repair and regenerate tissues, fight infections and cancer, and relieve pain and inflammation[148].

Depending on the light wavelength and frequency, mitochondria can heal, stem cells are activated and microbiome imbalances can be corrected[149]. Blue light inhibits the replication of infections, including parasitic and bacterial infections, augments immune function and reduces inflammation[150]. Red light is anti-inflammatory to tissues and modulates the nervous system for pain relief[151]. Full spectrum light reduces seasonal affective depression[152], and Ultraviolet light therapy helps improve symptoms of eczema[153].

The regenerative therapies I have described above help slow down the aging process because they are designed to impact the function and health of your cells. As you become more youthful at the cellular level, you begin to manifest youthful appearance naturally, without looking like superficial robots. These regenerative therapies accentuate your inner and outer beauty and radiance in a natural way.

At this stage, regenerative therapies can increase longevity and wellbeing and help you function optimally. You feel stronger, healthier, more vibrant, more functional and more motivated to be creative. Your capacity has expanded. You naturally begin to create a new lifestyle, new daily routines, new skills, a new career, new relationships, and new opportunities for your personal growth.

You begin to create more joy. You are no longer burdened by the weight of toxins, emotional stressors and pain. You feel free mentally, physically, emotionally and energetically. At this stage, you naturally acquire a growth mindset, expanding yourself and recognizing your capacity to become joyful beyond your wildest dreams. And you are now ready for the next step of the KHOSH Method™: Relate to Elevate.

Step 6:

Relate to Elevate

"I slept and I dreamed that life is all joy. I woke and I saw that life is all service. I served and I saw that service is joy."

Kahlil Gibran

A case report published in 2023 showed that six women who underwent an eight-week plant-based diet and lifestyle transformation, along with supplementation, reversed their internal age by an average of 4.5 years within two months[154], based on the Horvath DNAmAge clock. Although this was a small pilot study of relatively short duration, the study nevertheless suggests the power of dietary and lifestyle changes with supplementation to halt aging.

Now, imagine what would happen if the study incorporated meditation, prayer, reflection and this sixth step of the KHOSH Method™: relate to elevate. When we relate to others, when we are authentic in our relationships, when we trust and are trustworthy, when we love and accept love, when we are respectful and courteous, when we approach others with a smile and genuine kindness, giving them our time and focus, our spirit is elevated. We create joy for ourselves and others. We elevate ourselves as we relate.

Relating to others requires us to approach our relationships and work from a place of joy and service. It is about recognizing that the more we genuinely serve others, the more joyful we become. Our work becomes a form of service and service a form of worship.

Joy (khosh) is like a boomerang – the more you give it away, the stronger it comes back to you. This process of giving to others and not expecting to receive back often provides us with spiritual strength and blessings. During this sixth step, it is important to build authentic service-oriented relationships with others, and a strong relationship with your Creator or the Greater Universe through your own essential tools and spiritual practices.

As humans we have been endowed with the faculty of meditation, which informs and strengthens our spirit. 'Abdu'l-Bahá said in his talks in Paris in 1912: "Meditation is the key for opening the doors of mysteries. In that state man abstracts himself: in that state man withdraws himself from all outside objects; in that subjective mood he is immersed in the ocean of spiritual life and can unfold the secrets of things-in-themselves. To illustrate this, think of man as endowed with two kinds of sight: when the power of insight is being used the outward power of vision does not see."

During your meditation, remember your parents, grandparents, and ancestors. Remembering them with love, honor and gratitude helps maintain purity and cleanliness within your ancestral lineage, thereby reducing the spiritual baggage you may carry. When you pray for your parents and ancestors, and for the babies who were miscarried or aborted, you are providing a selfless act of service to them – and that service brings blessings to you. It elevates your cellular vibration to that joyful frequency of 528Hz we learned about in Chapter 15.

I draw your attention to the quote by the poet and writer Kahlil Gibran: "Your living is determined not so much by what life brings to you, as by the attitude you bring to life; not so much by what happens to you as by the way your mind looks at what happens."

Building Community

Relating to elevate not only involves building relationships with yourself, your family and colleagues, your ancestors, and your Creator, it also involves building community and acting responsibly towards your environment. Building community through acts of service, through praying and meditating together, through sharing meaningful conversations with each other, and through showing kindness to strangers, elevates your spirit while creating an environment of unity and oneness.

It is that oneness that elevates your soul further towards joy and youthfulness. By unleashing your feminine qualities such as being nurturing, gentle, intuitive, caring and kind, you begin to relate to others at a deep and inspirational level, which brings inner fulfilment and joy.

You forget your chronological age. You transcend the limiting mindset of aging. You gain capacity. Your mindset and soul expand. Your spirit elevates. And that joy and fulfilment, which is expansive and builds further capacity, reduces the stress within your body and your cells, while promoting cellular regeneration and DNA healing[155]. This type of expansive joy promotes wellbeing and longevity. It propels you forward towards graceful aging as you become an agent of transformation for others.

Finding your purpose

As you exercise and develop your feminine qualities and virtues, as you reflect and meditate, and as you connect with others and the Greater Universe, you will find your own individual higher purpose. That purpose is what gives you reason to continue to age gracefully. It gives your life meaning. It tells your cellular engine to keep on going.

It is that meaningful purpose, combined with deep inner joy, faith and courage, that continually propels you towards longevity – one that I hope is purpose-driven, unifying, world-embracing, resilient and positively transformative. You have been given only one beautiful chance to journey through this world as a woman.

Remember, no one leaves this world alive. The choices we make to become healthier and happier are not meant to stop us from dying, but to help us live a fulfilling life and to remain vibrant and healthy until our time is up. They help us achieve our purpose.

The Golden Gate Dr. Nooshin Khoshkhesal Darvish

Your life is your journey. You may choose to follow through these six KHOSH steps, or seek another route towards wellbeing. Nevertheless, it is up to you to mindfully choose your life's journey and to find the purpose that unlocks your best and most joyful life.

The mindful choices we make during our journey in this world of matter are to help us arise as Golden Gates, to attain our capacity, especially our spiritual capacity, to serve humanity, and to make the world a better place for each other and for future generations.

So, live your potential as a Golden Gate. Be a woman in every way in your own right.

"Khosh baash!"
I dare you… Be a Golden Gate!

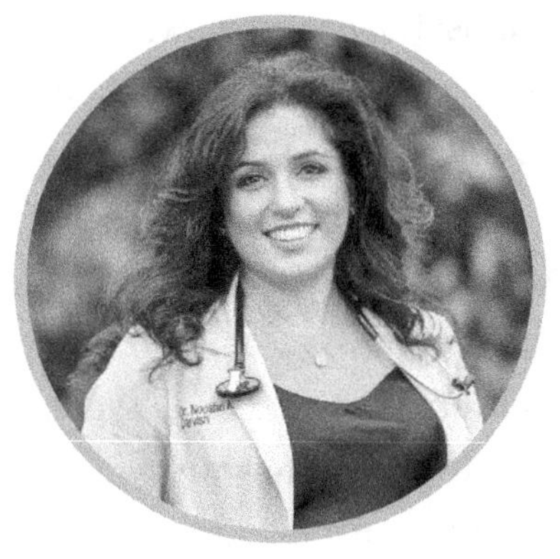

Biography

Dr. Nooshin K. Darvish, ND, ABAAHP

The Golden Gate Dr. Nooshin Khoshkhesal Darvish

Dr. Nooshin Khoshkhesal Darvish, an award-winning, internationally sought-after licensed naturopathic regenerative physician, is the founder and Chief Medical Officer of Holistique Medical Center in Bellevue, Washington. She completed her Bachelor's degree from the University of British Columbia, Vancouver, Canada prior to earning her Doctorate in Naturopathic Medicine from the internationally renowned Bastyr University in Seattle, Washington in 1995. Dr. Darvish completed a two-year residency in Naturopathic Family Medicine, has post-graduate fellowships in Integrative Cancer Therapies and Metabolic and Nutritional Medicine and is board-certified as a Diplomate in Anti-Aging Medicine.

Dr. Darvish holds an affiliate faculty position with Bastyr University, training resident physicians and medical students. She holds advanced training certifications in multiple therapies such as Regenerative and Stem Cell therapies, SOT (specific oligonucleotide therapy), Bio-identical hormone therapy, Ozone therapy, mistletoe therapy, and Platelet-rich plasma injection therapies.

As a Bahá'í, her guiding principle has been to harmonize the science of medicine with the art and spirituality of healing. As such Dr. Darvish's life purpose continues to be to 'Transform Lives from Within' and to serve through educating and healing the mind, body and spirit by practicing a perfect blend of the art and science of medicine.

She is the host of the Holistique Health Hour Podcast, a writer and editor for peer-review medical journals, has been interviewed on several podcasts and radio shows and speaks at international and national medical conferences.

As part of her continued humanitarian work, Dr. Darvish currently serves on the Board of Directors of the Mona Foundation. She is married and has raised three Golden Gate daughters. She loves to create, heal, dance, and travel.

GoldenGateBook.com 

Acknowledgments

ACKNOWLEDGMENTS

I have to take a moment to express my gratitude for those who have supported me, educated me, guided me and loved me during the past 54 years.

First and foremost, I am deeply grateful to and honor my late parents, Nahid Varqai Mazkouri and Arastoo Khoshkhesal, whose sacrifices, guidance, love and support led me to write this book as a tribute to their life of service and as a tool to help transform the lives of countless souls.

I honor all my ancestral grandparents, especially Bibi Ridvan, my maternal great-grandmother, who has played a pivotal role as a spiritual guide directing me towards carrying on the work and service she began 100 years ago as a healer and physician.

To my loving sister Negin, my wise brother Nabil and their spouses, Behnam and Mahsa, thank you for your love and support.

To my three beautiful and powerful Golden Gate daughters, Sanna, Maleka and Delbar who continue to teach me, love me, propel me to be the best version of myself and bring me so much joy - THANK YOU! I am deeply grateful to each of you and am utterly blessed to be your mother.

And thank you especially to my beloved husband Jahanshah for your continual love, patience, guidance and support. Thank you for the learning moments and the teaching opportunities, the challenges and the in-depth heart-to-heart conversations, your continual guidance and unconditional love, and the eternal soul connection. You provide me with a safe, comfortable, open and encouraging environment, enabling me to be inspired, to share, to grow, to learn, to be curious, to research, to create and to be me. Thank you for loving me no matter what, for pushing me beyond my comfort zone, for helping me elevate, and for always believing in me and for making me laugh. I am eternally grateful to you.

My mentors and educators, colleagues, Holistique Team and friends, there are too many to name but you know who you are: I thank you for all your continual guidance, encouragement, knowledge and leadership.

I am grateful to Charles Cooper and Himanshu Mehru for always being there to support me with technical support and to Cassidy Austin for organizing me and helping me launch this book.

With gratitude to my UK-based editor, Harriet Dennys, for shaping this manuscript I have been working on for ten years, my US-based content supporter and friend, Mariam Abdi Rowhani, for encouraging me to publish my life's work, to Barbara Vallini, for turning a basic word document into a book of art, and to Denise Cumella and her team at The Boss Books in Milan, Italy, for realizing my dream to publish this book as a service to humanity.

And, finally, I am grateful to Baha'u'llah, the Founder of my Beloved Faith, the Baha'i Faith, for constantly being the Light of my Guidance.

To learn more, access blogs and podcasts and contact Dr. Darvish, reach out to **https://drdarvish.com**

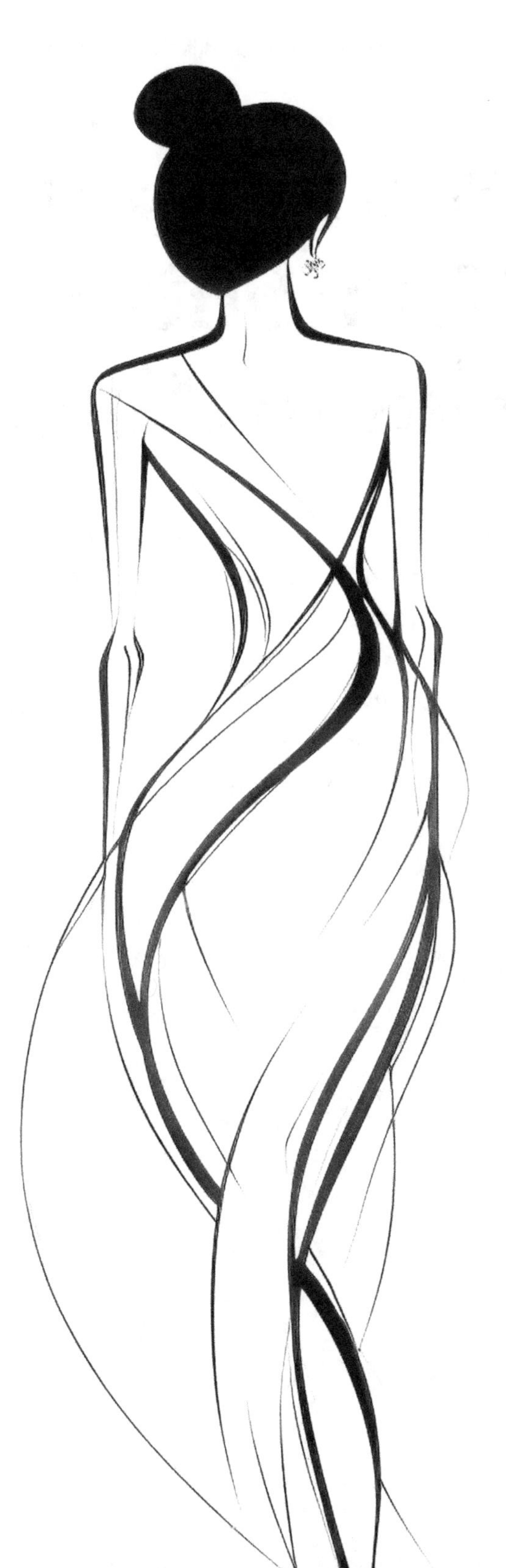

References and Further Sources of Information

Numerous references from respected scientific literature have been used in writing this book. These sources are acknowledged with a number at the relevant position in the text.

In order to save paper (there are over 480 cited sources), I have placed the corresponding details of – and links to – those studies on the webpage **GoldenGateBook.com/resources** so you can delve deeper if you wish.

Further Reading and Resources

For further reading material, bibliography and other helpful resources to support you in your healing journey, refer to GoldenGateBook.com/resources.

Appendix

APPENDIX A
The KHOSH Anti-Inflammatory Diet

Foods to Include
- Cruciferous Vegetables (e.g., kale, cabbage, brussels sprouts, arugula, broccoli, cauliflower)
- Squash, pumpkin, sweet potatoes, yams, purple potatoes
- Liver foods: carrots, beets, artichoke, lemon, lime
- Parsley, cilantro, leeks, green onions, red onions, garlic
- Cooked or warmed mushrooms (reishi, shitake, lions mane, bell)
- Organic Fruit: berries, green apples, green banana, pears, pomegranates, cherries, grapes
- Healthy fats: avocado, avocado oil, olives and extra virgin olive oil, 100% grass-fed ghee, coconut oil
- Seeds and seed butters (pumpkin, sesame, flaxseed, hemp seeds, sunflower seeds)
- Cold water wild fish: salmon, sardines, herring, mackerel, anchovies
- Occasional lamb
- Small legumes: mung beans, split peas, green beans
- Fermented veggies made in sea salt (sauerkraut, kimchi), tempeh, miso
- Organic dark chocolate with stevia, yakon or coconut sugar
- Occasional soft goat cheese
- Non-allergy nuts: cashew, pistachios, pecans, walnuts
- Sweeteners: yakon, stevia, monk fruit sweetener, coconut sugar, local honey
- Grains: sprouted quinoa, sprouted millet
- Organic dried fruit: dates, prunes, apricot
- Spices: turmeric, cumin, cardamom, ginger, saffron, cinnamon, fenugreek, black pepper
- Himalayan salt or trace mineral salt
- Reverse osmosis water
- Organic teas: green and black tea, rooibos, honeybush, chamomile, peppermint, lavender, turmeric, cinnamon, raspberry
- Organic mold-free coffee

Foods to Exclude
- Nightshade vegetables (eggplant, tomatoes, green/red peppers, potatoes)
- Sugar: brown, refined, syrups, high-fructose corn syrup
- Artificial sweeteners
- Food coloring
- Yeast, moldy foods, fermented foods
- Alcohol, wine
- Dairy from cow's milk
- Eggs
- Corn
- Gliadin/gluten (rye, oats, barley, spelt and wheat)

- Rice
- Beans
- Fats & oils: sunflower or safflower oil, vegetable oil, corn oil, soybean oil, canola oil, margarine, hydrogenated and trans fats
- Sodas, fruit juice, carbonated drinks
- Kombucha, fermented drinks
- Cookies, candy, pastries, cakes, ice cream
- Processed meats – hot dogs, bologna, prosciutto, sausages
- Red meat, chicken, turkey, pork, bisson
- Snacks: chips, crackers, pretzels
- Nuts: peanuts, peanut oil, almonds
- Fried foods
- Charred barbecue foods
- Processed sauces (teriyaki, red sauce)
- Gums and fillers
- Tap water
- Canned foods and drinks
- High mercury fish: tuna, halibut, swordfish
- Aluminum foil, Teflon pots
- Microwave use
- Tobacco, smoking, recreational drugs

Hydrotherapy methods to reduce inflammation
- Ice towel over area of pain or fever
- Constitutional hydrotherapy
- Wet sock treatment
- Contrast Hydrotherapy
- Cold water immersion
- Cold shower rinse
- Cold foot bath and hand bath
- Epsom salt bath

Plant or Mineral-based Anti-Inflammatories
- Homeopathic Arnica, T-Relief or Traumeel
- Drainage Remedies, e.g., Pekana Inflamyar, gemmotherapy, UNDA
- Omega 3 low mercury, non-rancid oils (fish, flaxseed, chia seeds, walnuts)
- Curcumin extract from turmeric
- Ginger
- White willow bark
- Rosemary
- Blackcurrant
- Berberine
- Borage oil
- Bromelain
- Evening primrose oil
- Sage

- Serrapeptidase
- Rosehips
- Billberry
- Green tea
- Garlic
- Olives and olive oil
- Boswellia serrata (frankincense)
- Cat's Claw
- Pycongenol
- Resveratrol
- Capsaicin (chilli pepper)

APPENDIX B
Ways to Replenish to Nourish

- Deep breathing exercises
- Exercise
- Ozone therapy
- Hydration with clean filtered water and electrolytes
- Hot herbal tea
- Oxygenation
- Hyperbaric oxygen therapy
- Cooked warm organic whole foods
- Sleep 7-8 hours a night
- Neutral temperature baths
- Essential oils
- Walk in nature
- Grounding: walk on grass with morning dew, or on beach
- Cuddle a loved one or a pet
- Hold hands with your partner
- Listen to your favorite soulful music
- Play with a baby
- Read a book or play a game
- Meditate, pray and reflect
- Gratitude journal
- IV Vitamin therapy and IV Hydration
- Vitamin, mineral, Essential fatty acid supplementation
- Bio-identical hormone therapy

APPENDIX C
Root Sources to Identify and Remove

Physical:
- Food sensitivities and allergies
- Environmental toxins
- Chemicals, glyphosate, pesticides
- Fluoride and other chemicals in water
- Dental amalgams, metal implants, fillings, other toxic dental materials
- Head injuries
- Hormone imbalance
- Stress
- Bacterial, fungal gut imbalance (dysbiosis)
- Mold and mycotoxins
- Metals
- Mineral deficiencies
- Digestive malabsorption
- Medications
- Supplements and fillers
- Vaccination adjuvants
- Infections: Bacterial, viral, parasitic, helminth, spirochete
- Stealth infections: in jaw/teeth, around scars, around implants
- Scars, piercings, tattoos
- Sites of physical trauma
- Spinal and extremity misalignments
- Mitochondria stress

Mental:
- Negative thoughts
- Perceived stress
- Obsessive thoughts

Emotional:
- Emotional attachments
- Grief, fear, guilt and shame
- Anger, resentment
- Loneliness, isolation
- Unworthiiness
- Powerless

Energetic:
- Electromagnetic/cellular
- Ancestral

APPENDIX D
Tools for Letting Go

Drainage:
- Liver, kidney, skin, lung, large intestine
- Lymphatic drainage, glymphatic drainage
- Drainage homeopathic remedies
- Dry brushing, trampoline jumping, walking, vibration exercise, massage
- Ionic footbaths
- Ondamed therapy
- Organic Whole Food
- Anti-inflammatory diet
- Plant-based diet
- Elimination diet
- Liver detox diet

Depuration:
- Sweat: sauna, bathing, exercise
- Breathe
- Enema or colonhydrotherapy
- Urinate
- Epsom salt baths
- Fasting
- Water fast
- Intermittent fast vs time-restricted fast
- Dry fast
- Juice fast
- Liquid fast
- Bone Broth fast

Detoxification:
- Supplementation for Phase I, Phase II and Phase III detoxification
- IV Therapy
- Anti-microbial therapy
- Chelation therapy
- Colonhydrotherapy
- Binders
- Emotional Release:
- ND Square
- EMDR
- EFT (Emotional Freedom Technique)
- Meditation and Reflection
- Journaling
- Humming, singing
- Brain spotting
- Ondamed biofeedback therapy

Ways to Support Depuration and Detoxification

- Deep Breathing exercises
- Clean filter water
- Get 7-8 hours of sleep
- Infrared sauna
- Epsom salt/baking soda bath
- Mud bath
- Hot and cold water therapy
- Fasting
- Exercise
- Dry brushing
- Enemas
- Colon hydrotherapy
- Minimize pharmaceutical medications whenever possible

APPENDIX E
Phase I Detoxification Foods

- Green tea
- Black tea
- Rosemary
- Fish oil
- Chicory root
- Algae
- Salmon
- Astaxanthin
- Turmeric
- Curry powder
- Cruciferous vegetables
- Resveratrol

Phase I Detoxification Botanicals

- Quercetin
- Broccoli
- Kale
- Rosemary
- Garlic
- Fish Oil
- Chicory root

Phase II Detox Foods

- Cruciferous vegetables
- Resveratrol
- Citrus
- Dandelion
- Rooibos tea
- Honeybush tea
- Soy
- Ellagic acid from berries, pomegranate, grapes, walnuts and blackcurrants
- Ferulic acid (from whole grains, roasted coffee, tomatoes, asparagus, olives, berries, peas, citrus)
- Turmeric
- Curry Powder
- Astaxanthin

Foods to Increase Cellular Glutathione

- Cruciferous vegetables
- Allium vegetables (chives, garlic, leeks, onions)
- Resveratrol
- Garlic
- Citrus
- Fish oil
- Black soybean
- Purple sweet potato
- Curcumin
- Green tea
- Rooibos tea
- Honeybush tea
- Ellagic acid
- Rosemary
- Ghee (clarified butter)
- Genistein
- Fermented soy (miso, tempeh)

Nutrients to support Glutathione and Detoxification

- Vitamin B6 – Turkey, chicken, amaranth, lentils, pistachio, sunflower seeds, prunes, and garlic
- Magnesium – Nuts, seeds, beans, whole grains
- Selenium – Brazil nuts, turkey, lamb, chicken, eggs
- Methionine – Turkey, chicken eggs, beef, brazil nuts, soybean, spirulina, sesame seeds
- Cysteine – Turkey, pork, chicken, eggs, soybean, spirulina, sesame seeds, oats
- Glycine – Turkey, pork, chicken, amaranth, soybean, peanuts, pumpkin seeds, beef
- MethylFolate (L-5MTHF) – Mung beans, adzuki bean, legumes, liver, sunflower seeds, quinoa, spinach, asparagus, avocado, mustard greens, artichokes, spinach
- Alpha-lipoic acid – Spinach, broccoli, tomato, peas, Brussels sprouts, visceral meats
- Functional foods – Turmeric, milk thistle, artichoke, cruciferous vegetables

Amino acids used in phase II conjugation and selected food sources

Glycine
Turkey, pork, chicken, soybean, seaweed, eggs, amaranth, beef, mollusks, peanuts, pumpkin seeds, almonds, duck, goose, mung beans, sunflower seeds, lentils, lamb, bison, lobster and fish

Taurine
Many cooked meats and fish supply taurine. Taurine is also synthesized in the body from cystine (requiring niacin and vitamin B6) and homocysteine (requiring additionally betaine and serine)

Glutamine
Plant and animal proteins such as beef, pork, chicken, dairy products, spinach, parsley and cabbage

Ornithine
Ornithine is synthesized endogenously via the urea cycle, requiring arginine and magnesium

Arginine
Turkey and pork are especially rich sources, also chicken, pumpkin seeds, soybean, butternuts, egg, peanuts, walnuts, split peas, mollusks, almonds, sesame seeds, lentils, fava beans, mung beans, pine nuts, beef, sunflower seeds, and white beans